Burn Bright, Not Out

Burnout Solutions for Nurses in a Broken System

GIOVANNA NAVARRO, RN, BSN

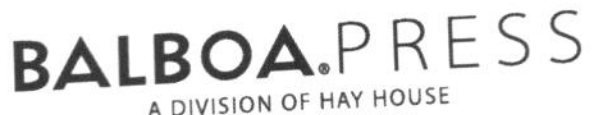

Balboa Press books may be ordered through booksellers or by contacting:

Balboa Press
A Division of Hay House
1663 Liberty Drive
Bloomington, IN 47403
www.balboapress.com
844-682-1282

Because of the dynamic nature of the Internet, any web addresses or links contained in this book may have changed since publication and may no longer be valid. The views expressed in this work are solely those of the author and do not necessarily reflect the views of the publisher, and the publisher hereby disclaims any responsibility for them.

The author of this book does not dispense medical advice or prescribe the use of any technique as a form of treatment for physical, emotional, or medical problems without the advice of a physician, either directly or indirectly. The intent of the author is only to offer information of a general nature to help you in your quest for emotional and spiritual well-being. In the event you use any of the information in this book for yourself, which is your constitutional right, the author and the publisher assume no responsibility for your actions.

Print information available on the last page.

ISBN: 979-8-7652-5839-2 (sc)
ISBN: 979-8-7652-5838-5 (e)

Library of Congress Control Number: 2024926132

Balboa Press rev. date: 02/19/2025

Disclaimer

Some names in this book are real, while others have been changed to protect individuals' privacy.

This book is intended to provide information and insights on overcoming and recovering from nurse burnout based on personal experiences and professional knowledge. It is not a substitute for professional medical treatment, psychological consultation, or evaluation. Readers are encouraged to seek professional advice for any health-related issues or concerns.

Contents

Praise for *Burn Bright, Not Out*

Giovanna's book is a transformative guide for anyone struggling with burnout. Through raw and honest accounts of her own journey, she builds a foundation of trust and relatability, seamlessly leading readers to a practical, evidence-based, step-by-step program for lasting change. Her unwavering support and compassionate approach shine through every page, making it feel as though she's right there beside you. This isn't just a book—it's a rare and invaluable companion for reclaiming your energy, purpose, and joy to truly live your best life.

—**Dr. Linda Bark**
Lifetime Achievement Award 2023,
Award-winning author, and founder of the
Wisdom of the Whole Coaching Academy

Giovanna is a globally experienced nurse with a huge heart who understands how to uplift others out of incredible stress. This book will be a much-needed healing for all the healers out there.

—**Ken Honda**
Bestselling Author of *Happy Money* and *True Wealth*

Author's Note

As a nurse with over 25 years of experience in critical care, including 8 years focused on neuroscience, behavioral health, and change management, I've dedicated my career to caring for others. However, it took a personal journey through burnout, autoimmune disorders, leaving bedside roles and coming back three years later, dealing with divorce, pregnancy, and foreclosure all at the same time, and finally, self-discovery to realize that I needed to focus on my well-being. I learned the hard way that I can't consistently have the energy, focus, and passion to pursue my dreams if I don't first take care of myself, no matter how much I want it to happen. Taking my well-being into my own hands was the starting point of my burnout recovery.

My journey through burnout and the subsequent discovery of holistic healing tools taught me valuable lessons I now feel compelled to share. I am uniquely positioned to address burnout because I can relate to the daily struggles we face in this profession—mastering subtle interventions, advocating for others, and working with a strong medical and scientific foundation. While doctors are equally knowledgeable and trained in complex medical conditions and procedures, their challenges can be different. For example, some may be less open to psychological approaches, which is concerning given the high rate of PTSD among healthcare professionals.

It all began when I experienced severe burnout while working as an electrophysiology lab nurse in a magnet hospital, followed by a divorce while pregnant. This unexpected turn led me to explore other venues, such as working in medical clinics and remotely as a care manager. I recovered from most consequences of burnout, but to my surprise, seven years later, my chronic anxiety worsened. Then depression hit, despite living what I thought was a healthy lifestyle and having a loving family environment at home. My current husband begged me to see a doctor, so I finally set aside my ego and went. I am fortunate to have an open-minded primary care doctor who listened. After lots of testing and follow-up visits, she determined that I was experiencing burnout again, along with a diagnosis of Sjogren's syndrome and possibly Lupus.

When I was struggling the most with autoimmune flares, I took full control of my life instead of doing what society expected. I embraced my new lifestyle instead of feeling angry about being sick. I stopped exercising six days a week and adopted a less strenuous routine, pairing it with a daily meditation practice. I followed an anti-inflammatory diet, took certain supplements, and small breaks throughout the day, no matter how much work was pending. Forcing myself to take breaks was the hardest part. No more multitasking, long hours working, or sleeping less than eight hours each day. Was my house clean every day? No. Did I complete all the tasks I had set for that day? No. Did I disappoint some people by not saying yes to everything? Probably. But guess what? The world didn't end. I felt and looked better than ever. My kids grew up to be healthy and happy teenagers, and I'm still happily married. Ha!

The second time around, I faced even more numerous challenges, from physical symptoms like joint pain and severe fatigue to mental health struggles such as mental fog, emotional exhaustion, and insomnia. However, these challenges also led to profound realizations about the interconnectedness of mind, body, and spirit and the importance of self-care. I incorporated tailored strategies during my breaks that I had recently learned from holistic approaches to health and wellness, including functional medicine. I discovered Dr. Joe Dispenza, who taught the scientific aspects of meditation, culminating in a three-year journey of recovery and transformation without the need for immunosuppressant medications with concerning side effects.

Feeling rejuvenated, grateful, and convinced that life doesn't have to be as hard as we've been led to believe, I became passionate about sharing my journey and the knowledge I had gained. I realized that healing isn't limited to just Western medicine recommendations. It's a multifactorial approach. This new perspective inspired me to specialize in behavioral health strategies, focusing on neuroscience, psychology, heart rate variability, and digital health. I became one of the first 500 board-certified nurse coaches (NC-BC) in the United States and the lead research nurse for a company that performs research studies nationwide, exploring the link between mental and physical well-being in partnership with the University of San Diego, the University of Texas, and Stanford, among other institutions. I also became a certified corporate consultant, personally trained by Dr. Joe Dispenza, conducting neuroscientific workshops for companies and their leadership teams around the world.

Three years ago, I found a mentor in Ken Honda, who taught me invaluable Japanese lessons about living a fulfilled and truly wealthy life. Working closely with him as a copywriter and customer experience specialist for his followers in the USA, I gained new insights into energy work, our relationship with money, how it intertwines with personal growth and happiness, and some Zen principles. This experience, combined with my strong medical and neuroscientific background as a nurse, deeply influenced my approach to how I train and coach my clients. I'm also actively involved with the Commission for Nurse Reimbursement to transform how nursing care is valued and reimbursed.

This book explores themes of holistic health, change management, and the power of lifestyle adjustments, alongside scientifically proven approaches to overcoming physical and mental challenges like burnout.

I am grateful to my family, and mystical friends who supported me through this journey. Special thanks to Barbie Kalev, Dr Joe

Dispenza, and Ken Honda for their mentorship and guidance, which helped shape my understanding of a fulfilled life.

I invite you to join me on this journey of discovery and healing. Let go of the fear, trust in the journey, and watch how your life improves. May this book inspire you to focus on your well-being and find balance, wealth and ease in your life.

In joy and gratitude,

Giovanna Navarro

RN, BSN
Board-Certified Nurse Coach (NC-BC)
Certified Corporate Consultant (NCSC)
Heartmath Certified Trainer and Trauma Sensitive Certification (HMCT)
Lead Research Nurse
Stress Management Specialist
HCA Caregiver of the Year Award Recipient, 2005.

Introduction

Burnout among nurses has reached unprecedented levels. Many nurses are reporting feeling drained emotionally. As we grapple with these statistics, first-line managers struggle to retain nurses. Patients don't always receive the care they deserve due to poor staffing ratios, adding even more pressure on nurses.

An important question emerges: **Who is addressing the healers' wounds?**

There's not a clear-cut solution right now for what we are experiencing. The solutions aren't arriving fast enough.

This book journey isn't merely an exploration; it's a call to action.

Nurses, it's time to take charge.

We are past the search for motivation and into finding practical solutions.

Important conversations are happening about the challenges nurses face with stress and burnout on different platforms. Many suggestions focus on improving our healthcare system and work environment, which are the main factors. However, my main concern is how nurses currently struggling can get the support they need right away. Many of us feel overwhelmed and need better tools to manage these challenges quickly.

Spending most of your time off recuperating from work is not fair to you or your loved ones. Well-being programs that ignore the root causes of burnout can feel like a frustrating dance—two steps forward, one step back.

Similarly, first-line and upper-level managers are struggling with their well-being. They are blamed for all the departmental issues. They feel lonely and misunderstood. Their hands are tied when wanting to advocate for their team and use their skills and autonomy. By making this change, organizations can achieve lasting transformation without breaking the bank. But getting there will take a few more years.

So, who will take care of you in the meantime?

We know that stress is a normal reaction to daily pressures. It can become unhealthy if it disrupts our daily lives. Some don't know that stress is emotional unease. Yes, your mental and physical responses also play a part. But it is the unmanaged emotions that give them energy.[1]

It doesn't make a difference if it's minor things like not having your favorite coffee or intense changes like ending a relationship. Your perception of something, even if it's not real, has the same effects. Let's say you're wide awake at night thinking of the worst possible scenario—the effects of stress on the brain and body are the same. These are actually physical reactions to negative emotions.

Burnout is the stress that you never recovered from. It's the result of an incorrect way of dealing with the chronic stress you have been exposed to excessively. Which generates emotional exhaustion.[2] Therefore, recognizing your primary stressors is fundamental to preventing or overcoming burnout.

This book is designed to increase your awareness of personal challenges, making it easier for you to identify what is actually stressing you out and why. It offers immediate strategies to prevent or mitigate the effects of chronic stress. You'll gain an understanding of the neuroscience behind behaviors and mental processes when transitioning from what we feel to how we express it. It provides language and meaning to the biological responses occurring within you, especially in the face of ongoing stressful situations. Because that's when it matters—when things are hard. From there on, everything else will be easier.

Let's be real; navigating this career is like trying to find a needle in a haystack, and we could all use a lot more support and guidance along the way!

Since we all love data, research, and facts, I'll share those with you throughout the upcoming chapters. My goal is that this newfound knowledge will spark your curiosity and inspire you to explore new perspectives, feel ready to ask the right questions and act accordingly.

Feeling burnt out doesn't mean you are not a strong nurse or that something is wrong with you. Our profession is facing unprecedented challenges from many angles. Overwhelming stressors call for proactive steps and exploring new approaches. In the upcoming chapters, we'll discuss why taking action now is important, even if you're one of the few not currently experiencing burnout.

Recovering from burnout may seem daunting. The truth is that nursing is a hard job, but hard is personal. The difficulty of the job depends on your unique situation. One day, you're worried about starting an I.V. The next, it's about doing chest compressions or protecting yourself from a violent patient.

We will explore ways to help you even if your work environment doesn't change.

My focus will be on solutions tailored to nurses in all fields and positions. From the bedside nurse to those working remotely, while recognizing that each of us understands our needs best. Now, I'm not here to sugarcoat things. You are here because something propelled you. As a nurse, something wasn't entirely satisfying you, and that's a good thing.

Growth is constant. Successful people are always curious and open to learning and adapting. It's not about knowing but also about applying that new understanding.

Reject the notion that sacrificing health or quality time is the norm. Break free from the assumption that *exhaustion is a badge of honor,* and let's start a journey toward a healthier, more fulfilling nursing career.

You are born with all the tools to shape the life you want and deal with any situation without letting it bring you down. I will show you how to tap into your inner wisdom and maximize it.

Readers will perceive these challenges in various ways, influenced by their belief systems. I want to provide insights beyond the usual story. After navigating through the content with an open mind, if you find that your answers aren't clear right away, don't worry. The goal is to equip you with the ability to pose new questions down the road that will help you move forward.

To get the most from this guide, adopt this mindset as you read each chapter: "How can I use this info to transform my life?"

These pages will provide your toolkit. "Burn Bright, Not Out" will give you a boost in strength, self-advocacy, and well-being. As you start this exploration, discover a roadmap to a more gratifying professional and personal life, including better financial wisdom. You already work hard enough; you deserve to get properly rewarded. It's time to focus on your health, happiness, abundance, and fulfillment – and this companion is here to show you how.

Your well-being matters. Start now, right here, with yourself. Your future in nursing deserves a proactive advocate—be that advocate for yourself.

01 From Dedication to Depletion

Another day of driving home, trying to keep it all together… holding back the tears and the burning frustration. When I get home, my loved ones deserve to see me calm and satisfied. I don't want to worry them by witnessing my exhaustion, stress, and overwhelming feelings. If they only knew what I go through each day. The expectations from everyone weigh heavily on me.

– MELISSA, RN

Does this sound familiar? Many of us, as nurses, struggle with this daily battle between professional demands and personal life.

- Are tasks that once brought you joy, now sources of discomfort?
- Is your confidence plummeting?
- During your time off, do you lack motivation to do anything?
- Do you feel like your work takes up so much of your time and energy you have nothing left for family and friends?
- Can't sleep well? Yet you know it's not depression.

Burnout is a dreadful feeling caused by the breakdown of the mind's defenses against stress. This breakdown creates isolation and makes us feel that something in us is not right.

In this book, I aim to share stress's deeper effect on nurses and my journey, along with practical tips and insights based on my experiences, research, and the support I've provided to multiple clients over the years. By focusing on our health, happiness, and professional fulfillment, we can prevent burnout and recover from it without needing to stop what we're doing, take time off, or change jobs- unless we want to!

Let's link our struggles with the actionable advice in this book because burnout won't go away soon. As conditions get tougher worldwide, we're all more likely to experience it. Burnout can't be solved with a single intervention. It requires a holistic approach and sustainable techniques. To comprehend this phenomenon, we must trace its roots and history.

Burnout in nursing is a well-recognized phenomenon. Herbert Freudenberger first introduced the concept of burnout in 1974. His work, particularly in observing the effects of stress and exhaustion among workers in a free clinic for addiction, laid the foundation for understanding burnout. Originally rooted in slang related to chronic drug abuse, the term burnout likened the syndrome to a charred building, symbolizing the cost of high achievement.

While no single perspective explains burnout, most experts agree that it is a state of emotional, physical, and mental exhaustion caused by excessive and prolonged stress.[3] As nurses, we understand the many obstacles unique to our profession, from the high demands of patient care to the emotional toll of seeing suffering.

Body Talk

I believe that burnout is closely linked to how our bodies perceive and respond to our surroundings.

Have you noticed how an animal in a zoo, even after years of being there and knowing it's safe, is always on the lookout? Whenever they eat, even if they're separated from potential predators, they're on high alert for dangers. Our sympathetic nervous systems react similarly, with a major difference: even when there are no real threats, our bodies can still activate the fight-or-flight response by thinking about potential dangers.

Animals don't dwell on past events; they shake off the stress and move on. We, however, often replay experiences, holding onto those memories and the emotions attached to them. When we remember those events or encounter similar situations in the present, our sympathetic nervous system kicks in to protect us. This stress response is important for our survival—this instinct helps in the short term. But if we can't turn it off, stress becomes chronic and harmful, constantly activated without resetting.

This unchecked stress mechanism leads to burnout. Our parasympathetic nervous system, which helps us relax, recharge, and regenerate, can't do its job effectively if we're always in a state of perceived threat.

You might wonder how to turn off this stress response if it's innate in all of us. Being proactive about your well-being matters most when things are hard. It's not just when you're feeling good and motivated and everything is going well that you need to step out of your comfort zone—it's especially important when you're not, as I will explain in these chapters.

I know that stress and burnout affect everyone differently. I honor your and everyone's journey. By no means do I want to sound dismissive of what many of us have experienced, especially in healthcare settings. I've gone through it, and it was hard to find people who understood and supported me. However, there's something important you need to know that has been scientifically proven—it's not just wishful thinking.

Everyone can overcome challenges, despite their circumstances. In engineering, *soft technology* refers to processes like decision-making, strategy development, training, and concept formation—essentially, human-based technologies. We are all born with the hardware: our brain and our neural connections. They are necessary for success. Yet, some mental states, like our beliefs and perspectives, can make it challenging. Our mindset is our software. There is no problem with the hardware, but there are many problems with the software nowadays.[4]

So if stress is innate in us and our body gives us a stress response to keep us alive. It makes sense this goes both ways. Our body also gives us mechanisms to manage stress in a balanced way. Our stress levels shrink when we escape or solve the threat (person, predator, or perceived worries). And when we can't due to constant or pressing circumstances, it knows how to reduce it as well through emotional regulation.

This is our focus: *solving the threat we sense*. Most of us need to learn how to do it or how to do it consistently.

How you see stress and respond to it is important. Your current mental state will greatly influence how you respond to stress. How you go from feeling it to expressing it is key. It lets our body deal with stress well and not accumulate it.

When relaxed and/or resting, you renew all your biochemical systems. You are integrating and processing your recent experiences. You are recovering your energy levels, which is the *recovery mental state*.[5] Most of us know quality sleep is important, yet we often struggle with it for many reasons. I want to encourage you to prioritize it even more because numerous EEGs in research studies show that during deep sleep, marked by delta waves, the brain facilitates vital processes like repair, memory consolidation, and emotional balance.[6] This isn't just theory—there's biochemical evidence to back it up. I will share tools to help you improve your sleep in Chapter 5.

From there you can move on to be at your *maximum performance level*. Which is a mental state in which you are creative, efficient, and productive. Like when writing a book, making a painting, giving a public speech, or seeing patients in a calm environment. You are focused on the task at hand, and everything is flowing smoothly. Great leaders in schools, companies, and certain societies make sure most people are in this state of flow. So if your workplace also encourages this, cherish it because not all companies or managers have this mindset. If most people in an organization, school, or company are burned out, then something needs to be managed better. This is important to remember, especially in our current healthcare system.

Last, the third mode is the most common. It happens when you feel threatened by something or someone. Sadly, it is so frequent that it has become normalized, which is when you are in a *survival mental status*.[7] Your behavior reflects resistance mechanisms like attacking, avoiding, or feeling upset. These reactions have become so common that most people believe they're normal. As a result, they accept them as part of daily life, doing nothing about it even if they don't like it. They assume it's unavoidable.

Suppose the body constantly believes the person is in danger, whether it's from an immediate physical threat or the feeling of being judged. You might feel judged during a meeting, criticized by a friend or colleague, or worried about your future with the company. To your survival mechanism, it's all the same. The stress response gets activated regardless of the type or severity of the perceived danger. It's either on or off; there is no grey area. This was well described by Professor Walter Cannon in 1932.[8]

The stress response directs the body to focus on sending blood and nutrients to the muscles in the extremities rather than the brain, as the brain consumes significant blood.[9] Additionally, the body continues to release adrenaline, typically reserved for life-threatening situations. To make matters worse, you are jacked up with adrenaline, your heart is racing, ready to flee when, in reality, you are sitting in front of a computer. Your body struggles to reconcile this incongruity. Energy reserves are depleted even without physical exertion. You never got up from your chair but ended up physically, mentally, and emotionally drained. We experience exhaustion with minimal to no recovery time. Eventually, burnout sets in.

Someone burnt out doesn't get angry or defensive anymore - they're stuck. They've lost their will to overcome. Their mind gets stagnant and can't adapt. There's no fight left in them. There's no survival mechanism.[10]

So, if we know that it is not a structural problem and we also know that we have enough neurons and connections, then that means we just lack the right mindset. We are not in flow or recovery mode. It makes sense that we need to learn how to change our mental state at will and with a strategy.

A strategy that works if you apply it. When you shift your mind, you will convince yourself that there is a way out of burnout. Because it never was a structural issue, it is something functional. This awareness gives it a whole new meaning.

If not recovering after exercise leads to reduced stamina and performance, in the same way that burnout does on an emotional and productivity level, we can apply the same principles here.

Healthcare professionals burnt out hold valid concerns. It's unfair that they are in this difficult situation. It was never their fault, an unbalanced healthcare system caused this mess. Nurses need help finding a solution that works exclusively for them. Yet, they struggle to pick which one is the best for their specific situation because they have so many things coming at them at once. From the unapproachable doctors to the demanding family members, uncooperative coworkers, and violent patients. The list of risk factors for burnout never ends. They don't know which one to address first.

In addition, sometimes, there is a lack of financial tools to help us make informed decisions. We feel like we are not making progress in any area and wonder if recovery is even possible.

Let's explore this daunting question together. I will break it into segments. This will help you integrate the knowledge more easily. It will also help you rank which issue to solve first in the complexity of burnout.

Common Risk Factors for Burnout

Many people know that they feel bad. But they do not know whether it's burnout or something else. They have not yet found the common causes. So, let's review them here.

- The first factor is the lack of control. It is the perception that we cannot do anything to change what is happening.

Not having a say in how you do your job is one example. This can be about your schedule, patient assignments, or workload. Or, it can be not having what you need to do your job. These things can ruin your goals, your progress, and your productivity. Another problem is the lack of clarity. Your boss or others have yet to communicate their expectations to you. This makes it difficult to know if you're doing a good job. Understandably, this can create uncertainty about job performance. Many people of working age feel that hard work might not lead to better opportunities, and that's a concern we can address together.

- The second factor is a conflict of values. Ask yourself:
  - How do my boss, my team, and my organization make decisions and invest resources?
  - Do I feel good about those underlying motivations?
  - Are they aligned with what is valuable?
  - Do they seem open to change?

  This ambiguity makes you lose motivation to work hard and the desire to persevere. It makes you less productive and opens the door to procrastination at work or in other parts of your life. We are seeing more of this in healthcare. Unfortunately, healthcare organizations rank profit over patient outcomes and staff safety.

- Third, we have insufficient rewards. You push yourself hard to work, study, or complete a project only to find that there is no reward for trying harder. Or maybe there is but the reward for the job you performed doesn't match what you expected. The effort and time you put into them doesn't come close to what you received.

  This happens a lot for many healthcare professionals. Where the most efficient worker, instead of being fairly rewarded, is punished with more work because he can handle it.

In my case, I worked in the IMC unit, and it happened more than once. I would always get assigned unstable, septic patients all at once. They had many drips or were ICU overflows with bigger demands. When I asked my supervisor, she said it was because I was one of the few who could handle the stress and work demands. This created a huge conflict of values for me, tearful drives back home, and many sleepless nights. I didn't know what else I needed to do to enjoy my job and receive a better salary.

If greater effort is not associated with a greater reward, our brains quickly learn not to try harder. The brain chooses efficiency and avoids wasting energy on tasks that don't provide a return. This sense of insufficient reward is more noticeable today than ever, especially in the wake of the COVID-19 pandemic. The cost of living and workload have increased faster than salaries, leaving many feeling like their hard work isn't being fairly compensated.

- The fourth and most obvious trigger for burnout is work overload, especially tasks requiring immediate attention. Urgent matters significantly affect our brains and cortisol levels, far beyond a heavier workload alone. This holds true even when there's no specific deadline or time pressure. As nurses, we encounter this daily; each patient demands our full attention, regardless of the level of urgency. When our workload aligns with our capacity, we can manage tasks and still find time to rest. However, chronic overload prevents us from restoring balance.
- The fifth factor that triggers burnout is less modifiable, and it is fairness. Do you believe that you receive fair treatment? Does your work go unnoticed, or are you acknowledged for your efforts? Injustice and a bad work environment might

also mean not being able to work without stress. This can make burnout worse.

Now that we've explored the concept, it's clear: burnout happens when your daily tasks clash with your core values. You're likely to feel a loss of personal identity, causing you to lose touch with who you are and what you've achieved.

Distinguishing Burnout from Other Challenges:

To grasp burnout, we must distinguish it from other challenges. In the mid-1980s, there was a suggestion that a distinction should have been made between work-related burnout and clinical burnout. Some even questioned the most used burnout tool, the Maslach Burnout Inventory (MBI). Allegedly, it was not appropriate as a diagnostic tool for patients[11] Compassion fatigue, moral injury, and major depressive disorder share symptoms with burnout but have distinct core features. Several authors have warned against using the label *burnout* when the diagnosis is uncertain. This is because it risks providing inappropriate treatment or leaving depressive episodes untreated.[12]

Burnout is not a medical condition. It is an occupational phenomenon. Rachel O'Neill, PhD., emphasizes that burnout can serve as a door to much worse health issues if not properly addressed.

- Compassion Fatigue stems from continuous exposure to the traumas of others. It leads to emotional exhaustion and a reduced ability to empathize. It often affects those in caregiving professions, causing feelings of apathy or detachment.

- Moral injury is a psychological response. It is due to actions that violate an individual's conscience or morals. It results from seeing or participating in events that go against one's values. This causes distress and problems in the mind, actions, behaviors, and relationships. It can also harm the spirituality of the individual.
- Major depressive disorder (MDD) is a mental health condition that significantly impairs daily functioning and can only be diagnosed by a specialist, including psychiatrists, clinical psychologists, primary care doctors, and licensed mental health counselors. Persistent and intense feelings of sadness, hopelessness, and a lack of interest or pleasure in nearly all activities are the most common symptoms.

Fast forward to May 2019. The World Health Organization officially calls burnout a syndrome characterized by:

- Feelings of exhaustion
- Mental distance from one's job
- Reduced professional effectiveness

Reading about these characteristics might make it seem like burnout isn't a big deal. However, the reality is different. It's important to understand where a person experiencing burnout is coming from, how they perceive their world at the moment, and how they are coping with these three characteristics.

If burnout is a syndrome resulting from unmanaged stress, you need to know how to spot the signs and stop it in its tracks. There's no quick fix; you can't compromise your health and well-being while relying on your employer to address the issue, even if they are responsible for 90% of the risk factors associated with burnout. While Western medicine can temporarily alleviate severe symptoms, there's no magic pill. Entrusting someone or something else to solve the problem for you is unwise and can jeopardize your future in various ways.

Even if your employer decides to adequately staff your department, offer bonuses, and provide fair compensation tomorrow, the consequences of burnout won't vanish overnight. Your body will still require time to recover, mainly because we often experience all five common risk factors for burnout, as mentioned previously. Taking responsibility for your life and using specific tools tailored to your needs is essential before the situation worsens.

Consider this scenario: if a patient arrived with pronounced symptoms linked to the five most common risk factors for stroke, you, as a healthcare professional, would promptly take action. It's a no brainer for us. Why not adopt the same proactive approach in your personal life? Now that you're aware of these five risk factors affecting your well-being, it's time to focus on your health and put preventive measures into practice. Just as you would intervene swiftly to address a patient's health concerns, apply that same diligence and care to safeguard your well-being. Take charge of your health journey and make proactive choices to mitigate the impact of these risk factors before they escalate.

Navigating the Stages of Burnout

Remember Herbert Freudenberger? He not only introduced the concept of burnout. With clinical psychologist Gail North, developed a model depicting burnout's progression through 12 stages back in 1992.[13] The model of burnout outlines a progression from an initial compulsion to prove oneself through excessive work to total mental and physical collapse. The stages include neglect of personal needs, social withdrawal, behavioral changes, and ultimately, severe depression and burnout syndrome.

Here, I summarize these stages:

1. **Excessive Ambition:** The individual feels a compulsion to prove themselves, often driven by high expectations.
2. **Working Harder:** To meet their goals, they start working longer hours and take on more responsibilities, often neglecting breaks and rest.
3. **Neglecting Needs:** Personal needs such as sleep, nutrition, and self-care are increasingly ignored in favor of work.
4. **Displacement of Conflicts:** Problems and conflicts are not acknowledged. The individual might feel threatened, panicky, and jittery.
5. **Revision of Values:** Personal values are altered, with work becoming the central focus, often at the expense of personal relationships and hobbies.
6. **Denial of Emerging Problems:** They may deny that their high-stress levels are causing any issues, instead blaming external factors.
7. **Withdrawal:** Social withdrawal begins with the individual avoiding friends and family and relying more on substances or other forms of escapism.
8. **Behavioral Changes:** Noticeable changes in behavior occur, such as increased irritability, aggressiveness, and cynicism.
9. **Depersonalization:** A sense of detachment from oneself and from others develops, leading to a loss of empathy and connection.
10. **Inner Emptiness:** The individual feels empty and may engage in compulsive behaviors such as overeating, alcohol or drug use, or excessive spending.

11. **Depression:** Severe depression sets in, characterized by feelings of hopelessness, apathy, and a lack of enthusiasm for life.
12. **Burnout Syndrome:** The final stage is characterized by total physical and emotional exhaustion, potentially requiring medical intervention.

As nurses, we can experience multiple stages and symptoms simultaneously or blaze through them at the speed of light due to the unique stressors and challenges faced in a healthcare environment like:

- The misconception that exhaustion is a badge of honor. Fueled by the belief that more sacrifice equates to greater dedication.
- The guilt that stems from tirelessly working while feeling they're never doing enough for their patients and colleagues.
- Frustration, an unwelcome companion in the pursuit of perfection, adds to the weight.
- The false belief that nurses and doctors are born with mental toughness. That somehow they can handle every challenge and always know what's best for their wellbeing.
- A toxic workplace where micro-management or gossip is the norm. Nurses face more pressure when trying to set healthy boundaries. They fear criticism for thinking about leaving the bedside world. They also fear criticism for considering a career switch.
- The threat of physical or verbal aggression from doctors, patients, and co-workers looms large.
- The stigma around seeking mental health support and fear of being labeled as a sign of weakness.
- Unrealistic expectations, often beyond one's control, create a breeding ground for burnout.

As you can see, burnout in nursing is not just fatigue. It is not just saying, "I worked too hard and I'm tired." Burnout isn't merely exhaustion either. Not all professionals endure it, but many healthcare professionals do. And the stakes are high. We are the only professionals who could literally change the quality of life of a person or even end it if we make a mistake at work. It's a risk that we can't afford to take.

Can you now understand better? Burnout in nurses is not due only to chronic stress at work. It's due to a combination of factors, including lack of support, high levels of responsibility, and unrealistic expectations.

Burnout does not mean personal failure or inadequacy. It's got nothing to do with who you are as a person or as a nurse. Nursing burnout is a fight against many relentless challenges. But it's a fight that we can win when we make informed decisions and take evidence-based steps.

So yes, burnout is a syndrome that opens the door to many serious consequences. Relentless stress causes emotional emptiness, decreased motivation, and physical exhaustion. It also leads to a notable decline in performance and a growing lack of motivation to do things. The lack of motivation leads to the belief that we have lost our capacity to be good at what we do.

We start comparing ourselves to our past selves—when we were energized, motivated, curious, and eager to make a difference—thinking we could be more efficient if only we could get back to that state. But the truth is, we're still competent and productive. The chronic stress we haven't recovered from has simply left us tired in body, mind, and heart. It's like returning from a vacation only to feel like you need a staycation to recover from your time away.

You could have rested well for a few nights. You could have eaten balanced meals and had a regular exercise routine. But you still do not feel at your best, and everything seems uphill. It generates a poor quality of life if we don't stop the cycle. For most healthcare professionals, it's not whether we will face burnout but when.

Such exhaustion affects our mood. It makes us more prone to irritability, apathy, and impatience. It also makes us cynical. This harms our relationships with ourselves and others. It also affects our hormones, particularly those related to sex and sleep. It reduces our work performance.

Relaxing and recovering quickly is key. It lets you try again the next time a challenge arises. *Recovering from damage* and *avoiding further damage* are not the same thing. Now, I am talking about avoiding more damage.

Burnout significantly changes neural circuits, especially by activating the amygdala more intensely than other regions. This shift changes your perception of reality, making you more pessimistic and prone to negative moods. Physically, burnout leads to the growth of the amygdala and weakens its connections with the frontal lobe, which normally helps regulate the amygdala and reduce stress responses. These weakened connections create an exaggerated sense of risk, that leads to feeling more intense anxiety and fear, along with a decreased sexual desire, and less willingness to take risks necessary for personal growth and reward. Despite these changes, it's possible to rewire these circuits.[14]

Additionally, burnout doesn't just affect behavior and mood; it also affects attention. This complex interplay of changes underscores the profound effect burnout has on both the mind and behavior.

People with burnout might experience a reduced effectiveness of theta wave synchronization, thus negatively affecting hippocampal function.[15] Which is crucial for learning, memory processes, restorative tasks[16] and the control of complex behaviors.[17] Theta waves are often described as waves of *healing,* as the theta state is a period where the body and mind deeply relax and restore. This state enables the brain and body to rest and heal, while also encouraging learning, memory storage, and creativity. Reduced theta wave synchronization means a lower chance of entering the flow state. As I mentioned before, in the flow state, you are productive, with greater opportunities for creativity and excellence. A lack of theta wave synchronization can create a vicious cycle of poor productivity and worsening results.

Speaking of healing, in terms of diseases, it is important to be aware of this perspective. A person resists and says, "Why me, why did this happen to me?, I don't deserve this!". The immune system, which defends you from disease, cannot work as it should. It can continue to worsen if theta wave synchronization remains low.

But when a person turns why's into how's and says, "Look, I assume that this is my situation. I don't like it, I don't want it, I never asked for it, but I assume it. So from now on, I'm only going to focus on what I can do to change." The immune system is much more powerful and able to do its job homeostatically.[18]

As we close this chapter, it's key to acknowledge something. Though burnout classification for nurses may follow general models, we see it as a bigger deal that affects both us and our patients.

Understanding stress is the first step in solving burnout. In the next chapters, we'll look deeper at the impact of stress on nurses. We'll unravel the complexities of nurse bullying. We'll learn the knowledge needed to address the root cause of burnout for everyone.

If you're reading this book, you're ready to move past the pizza parties and massage chairs. You're now looking for real, practical solutions you can apply right away. It is possible but remember that this journey may have its ups and downs. Unpacking the layers of burnout can feel like exploring new territory, and it's normal to face obstacles along the way.

Some of you may find it tough to rethink long-held beliefs about dedication and sacrifice. Others might struggle with the societal pressures that contribute to the burnout story. I've faced these challenges myself more times than I can count.

As we dig into these issues, be prepared for moments of reflection. They might push you to rethink your current beliefs. The path to well-being isn't always a straight line. It takes bravery and commitment to break free from old habits. Remember, every challenge you face is also a chance for growth and positive change.

Our journey is not just about understanding burnout. It's about overcoming the hurdles that might hold you back from a better professional life. Join me as we face these challenges. Let's clear the way to a new sense of purpose and well-being.

Our legacy mirrors our dedication to healing—both for those we serve and for the healers themselves.

02 Can Stress Be My Ally?

"It's so hard driving home from work every day wondering if I'm really doing the right thing... If this is the field I'm meant to be in... or if I have a calling in something else that I don't know yet? I love being a nurse, but now I can't decide if I love it or LOVED it... if I need a break or what... and if I did leave this profession... where do I go next?... I wouldn't even know where to start. Some days are better than others, but I wanna love my job again like I used to & really feel like I'm making a difference because I don't feel like that anymore..."

– SARAH, RN

Sarah's words echo a truth many nurses face daily. If you've ever felt this way, it's a chance to reflect and consider how new coping strategies and a fresh look at your goals could help you navigate these feelings.

Stress impacts everyone differently, but for nurses, it can be overwhelming. The constant need to show empathy and strength, and be available for others can be challenging.

Despite the difficulties you encounter daily, they are often unnoticed. Your job involves working long hours, making quick decisions, and performing well under pressure. Unrealistic expectations and a lack of resources add to the stress, pushing you closer to burnout. Overcoming burnout may feel like a big challenge, but it is possible with the right support.

Reflect: Have you felt the weight of burnout? How has it affected you? Reflect on your experiences and consider the system's role.

According to Christine Sinsky, MD, vice president of professional satisfaction at the American Medical Association, burnout stems from the environment. It occurs when the workload and the resources for meaningful work don't align. She suggests that the best response to burnout is fixing the workplace, not the worker.[19]

I wholeheartedly agree, but what can you do in the meantime? Your patients can't wait—they need you now, strong, healthy, and fulfilled, and so do your loved ones.

Understanding Stress

To tackle burnout and improve your well-being, addressing the root causes is essential. Focusing on one cause won't solve the problem. Many factors contribute to burnout, as discussed in Chapter 1. Earning more money might help with low rewards, but it won't solve issues like excessive work, conflicting values, or lack of control.

Having the tools to address the root cause is key. *It all starts with choosing how to respond to stress.* Progress is only possible if you can identify the factors that trigger your stress.

Reflect: Have you identified the factors that trigger your stress?

How we respond to stress is personal. Everyone experiences it differently. Only you know what you're going through, how it affects you, and how stress manifests in your life. Today, knowing isn't enough. Understanding how stress connects to our world lets us develop strategies to solve burnout.

Stress in the nursing profession

Stress in the nursing profession is familiar, but did you know it can be a powerful tool to help you meet your goals? It's natural to react to life's challenges. Stress can improve performance, but too much stress can affect health and quality of life, leading to burnout.

The World Health Organization explains stress as feelings of worry or tension from dealing with tough situations.[20] Let's learn how to recognize and manage stress to make it work for us, not against us.

All types of stress, acute, episodic, or chronic, affect the mind and body similarly. Your body can't tell real threats from imagined ones. Whether it's a person, a financial issue, worrying about your next shift, or simply picturing worst-case scenarios, it's all the same to your body. Being in constant alertness drains your energy faster than you can replenish it.

Consider a quick example of how stress reactions are unique and important for nurses. When stressed, adrenaline helps us prepare for tough situations. For example, a nurse might quickly respond when a patient codes. We rely on training and experiences. Even if outcomes are uncertain, feeling confident in our efforts is important. So, yes, stress responses are normal and much-needed in our line of work.

Some individuals manage stress as their situations improve. In this scenario, the patient coded, the nurse acted accordingly, and she felt confident that she did the best that she could with what she had at that moment for that patient. She might feel empathy or sadness. But she can continue her work without carrying draining feelings like guilt or doubt. Practice and familiarity were key for this nurse in this example. Meanwhile, others adapt to ongoing challenges however they can. They do so, even if it affects their well-being. Since stress affects everyone differently, there isn't a one-size-fits-all solution. How we've balanced life's demands and our coping mechanisms shape our well-being. Balancing demands better requires consistency and familiarity as well.

The Effects of Stress on Your Body and Mind

Challenging situations, such as heavy workloads, money problems, or a fear of job loss, can trigger a rise in stress hormones. This rise affects your body and mind in various ways. At first, you might notice physical symptoms like a racing heart, headaches, muscle tension, rapid breathing, and fatigue. Emotionally, you could feel irritable, anxious, or impatient. Prolonged stress can cloud your thinking. It can affect your ability to focus and make decisions, which is important in nursing.

Reflect: What physical and emotional symptoms of stress have you experienced? How do they affect your daily life?

Unreleased stress builds up and makes individuals prone to overreaction. Even minor surprises, like not having the right tape at work, traffic jams, or family disputes, can trigger strong responses. The reason lies in the body's stress hormone levels. They stay elevated if people don't find ways to release that tension. They're more likely to develop more serious health problems. These include high blood pressure, chronic pain, arrhythmia, and inflammation among others.[21]

This increases the risk of systematic imbalances, autoimmune disorders, or blocked arteries. Recent studies have also revealed how chronic stress has a close relation to brain changes linked to anxiety, depression, addiction, and obesity.[22] People can also become less tolerant and resist considering others' ideas. They may become so focused on what's right in front of them that finding solutions and adapting to new perspectives can be harder. Eventually, this state of stress becomes the new norm. It's so familiar to your body that it becomes part of your identity.[23] Life can be challenging, and stress can consume individuals faster than they realize if they are not careful.

Nowadays, there's evidence that stress affects all stages of the disease process: genesis, progression, and recovery.[24] Also, it may be as bad for one's heart as smoking and high cholesterol.[25]

Reflect: What are your major stressors and which stress management strategies have you tried? What works best for you?

Have you ever noticed how dogs shake off stress?[26] There's a valuable lesson to learn from them. Keep following along for more insights!

Stress is a constant companion in the nursing profession, but it doesn't have to be your enemy. By understanding and managing stress effectively, you can turn it into a powerful ally. By getting clear on the action steps needed, we can avoid false starts or getting sidetracked.

Managing Stress Effectively

Remember our chat about the WHO's definition of burnout in Chapter 1? It's a syndrome resulting from chronic, unmanaged workplace stress.

Consider this: Imagine work is like juggling water bottles while balancing on a ball. What does it take to handle stress in the fast-paced world of healthcare?

Managing stress is about finding balance. It's not about eliminating stress entirely but learning how to make it work for you. There are two common ways people manage stress.

Distress hits when stress overwhelms us *because we don't know the outcome* of whatever we are dealing with at the moment. This uncertainty causes an imbalance. On the flip side, eustress is a good kind of stress. It comes from tackling rewarding challenges, like working out, planning a fun trip, moving to your dream house, or giving a speech. It leaves you feeling accomplished, knowing that the tough journey is worth it.

Our emotions are terrible leaders, especially fear. So, the key to managing stress is how we decide to perceive the situation and our beliefs about the outcome. Based on this, our minds choose how to react to stress.

When you're chronically stressed, it can feel like you're all alone, with a huge weight on your shoulders. But remember that you're not the only one facing these challenges, and seeking support is a sign of strength, not weakness. I've done it more than once and have never been disappointed with the outcome. Once you train your body to respond in eustress mode, even while at work, you become immune to burnout. The journey ahead will help you understand how to do just that.

Main reasons for stress in Nurses

For now, let's loop back to that example of a patient coding. If a nurse feels they could have done better, doubts may linger after a shift. Those emotions come home with you, and the constant 'what-ifs' drive you to reflect, learn, and improve. That might seem like a good thing—after all, isn't striving to be better part of the job?

But here's the real question: how will you know when you've done your best and that you are good enough?

Now, consider your coworker who always complains. Maybe she's overwhelmed by past experiences, shaken by a difficult phase in her career, or struggling with the fear of not being valued. She might be carrying stress from years of unresolved burdens, leaving her in a constant state of fight-or-flight. How can anyone feel safe, rested, or ready to tackle another day without a chance to reset?

These stressors—self-doubt, past trauma, lack of recognition, and chronic exhaustion—are part of a bigger picture. Reflecting on them can help you better understand your own response to stress, the challenges that many nurses face, and how you can foster a more supportive and compassionate environment. By recognizing these patterns in yourself and others, you can start to build stronger connections, encourage open dialogue, and create a workplace culture where everyone feels valued and supported.

Let's look at nursing through the lens of Maslow's hierarchy of needs and the stress rabbit hole. This will help you see that burnout isn't a personal failure; it comes from many factors coming together. By understanding these needs at your workplace, you'll gain insights into how strong and proactive you are. Many busy professionals in high-pressure jobs like yours use the tools shared here. They can transform your life and improve your well-being in a way that *aligns with your true self.*

Understanding Nursing Stress Through Maslow's Hierarchy of Needs

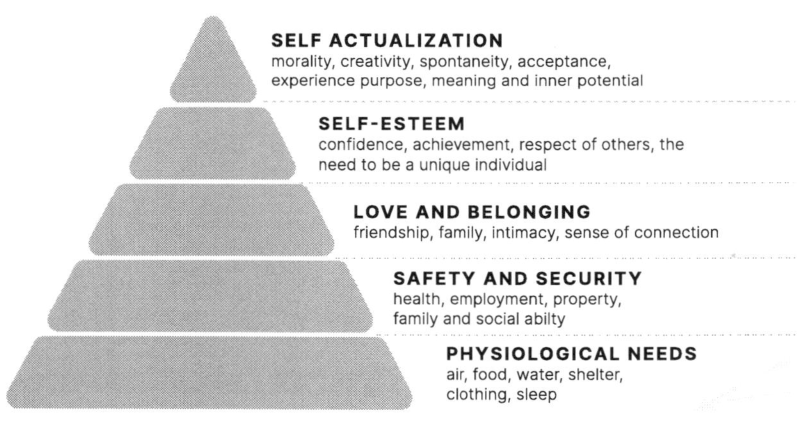

Maslow's theory helps us make sense of what drives us as people and as nurses. I mean, last time I checked, nurses are still human! We're more than just caregivers—we have feelings, hopes, and dreams, just like our patients.

- Maslow argued that the main need is for physical survival. It is the first motivator for behavior.[27] Our bodies need a few basic things to survive: air, food, sleep, and a place to call home. We have to meet these needs. They keep us healthy and focused, especially in the fast world of healthcare. Fortunately, you can meet most in a short period. As nurses, we see our clinical settings as dynamic. Let's think about:

How can you put your physical needs first, even amid the unpredictability? This will keep your body working well. Remember, the uncertainty could become an unmet need that causes distress.

- Safety and security give you peace of mind at work and at home. You'll feel more in control when you make your job more stable and predictable.

How do you navigate the challenges of the clinical setting to meet your safety needs? Do you have a strategy to help you maintain a sense of order and security amid the fast-paced nature of your job?

- Good friends are key. A strong support network outside of work is also super important for your happiness. Make time to nurture these relationships with your family and friends, and they'll enrich your life.

The desire for a sense of belonging can outweigh the need for safety in some individuals. This phenomenon may lead people to remain in codependent or toxic relationships. For nurses, this might show up as staying in a non-supportive workplace. Feelings of guilt about leaving co-workers might help decide here. I know that a work bestie makes a huge difference! If you work remotely, you still have concerns about patients and the issues you help them with. Also, the false belief that only hospital work is "real nursing" can affect these decisions. Nurturing our need for connection is important. I get it; I've felt that need as well. How can you satisfy this need healthily?

- Feeling good about yourself is important. When you face your self-doubts, you'll have better relationships because you can set healthy boundaries and enrich relationships that involve balanced give-and-take. You'll also have a clearer sense of direction.

Insecurity, as Maslow described it, includes seeing the world as threatening. This insecurity manifests as a lack of confidence, distrust, and fear of disappointment. If left unaddressed, it may lead to poor treatment of others and bullying. How might acknowledging and addressing insecurities about self-esteem and accomplishment influence your interactions with others?

- Doing work that matters to you is the key to a happy career. Chase growth while sticking to your values. Then, you'll find fulfillment. This experience is both exciting and unpredictable. I've experienced it for many years now. When I focus on something meaningful or joyful, my energy shifts. It brightens my mind and opens my heart. This brings a sense of lightness and brightness. Positive, creative thoughts flow. They align with my vision. The outcomes, though not always as expected, come together effortlessly. The right people, resources, and opportunities always appear at the right time.

How can you incorporate purposeful activities, creativity, and alignment with your values to unlock your full potential and experience growth and fulfillment in your life? Examples include serving others, exploring intellectual pursuits, having more spirituality, and connecting with the divine. Some also consider connecting with nature or mysticism a way to connect with their inner potential.

Understanding these needs can also give us a clearer image of what drives our patients and why they behave and react the way they do so we can have more meaningful connections and assertive communication with them.

Our needs vary throughout life, and our awareness and actions deeply influence them. Maslow believed that while meeting all needs at once may not always be possible, striving for fulfillment motivates us to experience peak moments. Being flexible with ourselves and letting go of perfectionism can reduce frustration.

Coping Mechanisms

Let's discuss coping mechanisms. Our bodies can handle short-term challenges well. In healthy people, both levels of cortisol and dehydroepiandrosterone (DHEA) increase in response to short-term negative emotions.[28] But when we struggle to meet our needs or face ongoing issues, for days or longer, we can resort to unhealthy ways of coping. Nurses and doctors do this to find quick relief from pain or stress, often thinking it's socially acceptable. However, these readily available methods can sometimes be harmful. We must remember that relying on these fixes can lead to behaviors that may not be helpful in the long term.

Coping mechanisms are influenced by various factors, including biology, psychology, and the environment. Social pressures also shape our coping strategies. For example, many people consider using social media on their cell phones a good way to relax. But it can take away time from more nourishing activities and become a difficult habit to break. This can make people feel they're not good enough by comparing themselves to what they see online, adding to their already lower DHEA:cortisol ratio, from dealing with chronic stress. This is a key biochemical marker of stress and accelerated aging,[29] along with the physical and physiological degradation I previously mentioned.

I was one of them. I used to go on social media without realizing how it affected my well-being and productivity. As I thought about it, I noticed I used it more during quiet moments, which made me feel more tired, and sometimes guilty. I spent so much time on my cellphone instead of having a nice talk with my loved ones or some much-needed quiet alone time.

Unhealthy coping mechanisms aren't a sign of weakness. It's nothing more than a sincere attempt by your mind to help you feel better. Once you know why they happen and their impact, you have a choice. Making changes and creating new habits requires self-awareness and embracing healthier alternatives. Please seek support from trusted friends, family, or professionals. They can help you navigate this process. Talking about it lets you develop new strategies, gain control over your emotional reactions, and build a strong support network.

Nurse Bullying

Recognizing the impact of low self-esteem is important for healthier interactions. When nurses bully, it's often linked to mental health and workplace problems combined with low self-esteem, insecurity, or a need for control.[30] Understanding why people bully can help support victims and empower bystanders to stand up to it and make things right confidently.

Research shows that some individuals who engage in bullying might battle conditions like depression, anxiety, or anger problems.[31] These issues often start from emotional neglect at home. Sadly, this behavior might get rewarded, especially when leaders don't step in. Bystanders who stay silent can unintentionally support the aggression. Those who bully may continue because they receive attention. When bosses give good reviews, it can perpetuate bullying if it's seen as being proactive.

Understanding this doesn't excuse the harmful actions. Instead, it helps reveal possible motivations. So, what's the solution?

1. **Boundaries:** Set clear and healthy boundaries instead of reacting with anger or frustration. Handling aggressive personalities with compassion and cleverness can take away their power because it shakes their control over the situation.
2. **Detach yourself:** Bullying has a lot to do with perceptions. It's more about the bully's insecurities and poorly managed frustrations than about you. Learn how to regulate your emotions and protect your peace instead of defending yourself impulsively. You must also express how you are feeling in a safe space with someone you trust. Don't hold on to them because it will drain your energy faster.
3. **Have a support group:** Bullies often run alone and may be less inclined to target a cohesive group. This strategy is effective in adult office settings.
4. **Stay informed:** Find out what measures are available at your workplace.
5. **Consider therapy:** For those who have experienced bullying situations, therapy can empower individuals by helping them realize they've done nothing wrong and enabling them to confront the bully.

If you have noticed bullying tendencies in yourself, it's okay! Everyone deserves a second chance. Recognizing it and deciding to do something about it is brave. Therapy, particularly cognitive-behavioral therapy (CBT), can be beneficial, especially if there are symptoms of depression.

I'll never forget when a client, a single mom of three, approached me just three months after starting her new job. Her male supervisor's constant bullying and harassment left her unable to sleep at night. She debated whether to stand up for her rights and risk losing her job or set an example for her three boys by setting healthy boundaries and demanding respect as a woman.

When she escalated the issue to HR, she was terminated. They didn't even try to hear both sides of the story.

This is a perfect example of what happens when leaders fail to address this behavior. It can become entrenched and even rewarded.

This needs to stop. Intimidation or humiliation should never happen to anyone, anywhere. No one likes a bully, and no one wants to be a bully, yet bullying is on the rise, even after all the organizational efforts to cultivate positive cultures.

So, why does it keep happening? Humans are complicated. Emotions, egos, power trips—mix them together, and you've got a recipe for disaster. Factors such as personality differences, feelings of superiority, power abuse, passive-aggressive behavior, and fear all contribute to the prevalence of bullying.

The consequences of workplace bullying are profound, including increased turnover, decreased productivity, and the creation of unsafe environments. The mental and physical health of those affected can suffer long-term repercussions.

Nurses, especially, get the short end of the stick. They face bullying from all sides—colleagues, patients, and families. Even in remote work settings, bullying can manifest through micromanagement via online interactions or emails. One nurse mentioned that doctors might use fear—a patient could die or have a bad outcome if the nurses do not do things properly—as a motivator to bully. Feelings of superiority and educational differences can also lead to bullying.

If upper management is responsible for up to 65% of incidents and you're in a position of power, it's time to step up and take proactive steps!

- Make it crystal clear that bullying won't fly on your watch. Show your commitment to a safe and healthy working environment by calling out inappropriate behavior to signal zero tolerance for bullying. Encourage employees to report bullying and treat every complaint seriously.
- Standing up for oneself may seem risky, potentially jeopardizing job security, so listening to your team's concerns and having open conversations can help you gain a better perspective and prevent complications down the road if the bullying doesn't stop.
- Beware of falling into the gaslighting trap, which can occur after confronting a bully. Put training programs into practice to educate staff about workplace bullying, respectful behavior, and positive conflict management. Additionally, collaborate with HR to ensure they are equipped to support you and your team effectively.
- Question whether the person is being bullied or simply struggling with workload dynamics or other stressors. Work overload or new systems that an employee doesn't understand or agree with might cause them to ignore protocols. Pay close attention to why an employee might be resistant to following orders.

"We live in the world our questions create."
-DAVID COOPERRIDER

Now that you have a greater understanding of how we generally perceive things on a deeper level and how we have adapted our behaviors to navigate the healthcare environment, can you see how the questions you ask shape your understanding and perception of the world? Asking the right questions can lead to deeper insights and uncover underlying issues.

As nurses, you've seen how amazing the human body can be at adjusting to challenges and staying strong. It works hard to keep you alive and healthy, even in the most extreme scenarios. You know this, but sometimes you forget to care for yourself. You put your health at risk by focusing on other things.

Sure, money is important. Self-care can be tough with all your responsibilities vying for attention. But if you don't take care of yourself, your health will suffer. When you're unhealthy, it's tough to be there for your loved ones and to enjoy life. So what's the point of working so hard if you can't even enjoy it?

Resistance to change and taking care of yourself holistically is a complex topic. To understand it, you need to look into your unique situation and the psychological barriers that hold you back. It's not a matter of willpower or a one-size-fits-all solution. Approach this with sensitivity.

I've coached people from all walks of life, and I've noticed a pattern: If a new behavior doesn't give you the same or better reward, you're less likely to stick to it. Changing a habit requires that you get something out of it, or you'll likely go back to your old ways. This is just how you're wired, so don't worry – you're not the only one who struggles with this. Some days still get the best of me!

Which is why I wanted to point out some possible scenarios briefly:

- Many of us know what we need to some degree.
- We understand why we need it, but most of us don't know how to achieve it sustainably.
- There is a common belief that the only way to succeed is by working hard, even if it means putting our needs last.
- Some of us feel the need to prove our worth daily. We keep comparing ourselves to other professionals and to the standards set by our parents and society about what makes a good and successful person.

The healthcare system often takes advantage of our good intentions. For example, it persuades us to take on extra shifts by appealing to our sense of duty and compassion for others. It may even throw in some puppy dog eyes from the manager. Many of us have fallen for it. Working from home has its own hurdles, including demanding expectations and micromanagement from some companies.

Yes, finding the root cause of why we don't focus on our health is key, but the right support is just as important. It's hard to make progress if we can't figure out what's causing our stress.

This chapter emphasized the need to understand the big impact of stress in general. Understanding how stress uniquely affects you as a nurse involves staying curious and asking the right questions instead of assuming it's the norm if many are in a similar situation. Embracing the constant changes and the pressure to excel is tough. They come from the demand for quick solutions in a rushed world. This path is definitely not for the faint of heart. If you don't have the right toolkit, you'll be fast-tracked toward burnout.

But here's the twist: beyond the daily demands, there's a truth we'll uncover – seeing stress as an ally. Turning the fear and worry you're experiencing into excitement and motivation can transform hard jobs into successful and enjoyable experiences.

Like when you treat a patient: if you know you can trust the medical equipment, you feel safe. Then, you can do what you do best: keep your patient stable. If you have the right tools for changing behavior, you feel in control. You can handle all the stress and surprises and stay in a state of ease.

I'll support you and guide you to tap into your inner wisdom and maximize your potential. Building resilience is one of the tools that can help you achieve this.

Yes, I said it – resilience! But hold on, don't make a run for it just yet! Hear me out.

I know that *resilience* might make some healthcare professionals cringe. But it's not about fixing you. You're not the problem – the healthcare system is. It's a flawed system and the root of the challenges you face. My approach puts you in the driver's seat. It gives you the tools to bounce back and succeed in a short period, no matter what obstacles come your way.

Rather than a burden or a sign of fault, think of resilience as one of the tools for safeguarding your well-being.

You can amazingly bounce back and grow, no matter what life throws your way. That's why being resilient is super important in your tough job. You deal with a ton of emotional and physical demands, so taking care of your mental health is key. It's like giving your mind a workout and keeping an eye on how you're doing. It's all part of the recipe for success in these challenging roles. I mean, even top athletes, the military, pilots, and cops use these tools – so why not you?

When you look at life from new angles, you see beyond the struggles and fires that need putting out. You'll discover a world of possibilities and achievable goals. Taking control of stress can be a huge weight off your shoulders. It lifts your mood, energizes your body, and keeps you healthy.

Stress can fuel your success. My own life is proof – I've harnessed its power and continue to enjoy it every day. By guiding many nurses through their darkest moments, I've learned what works. Now, I'm ready to help you too. Turn the page to discover the solutions that will unlock your full potential.

03 Challenging the Status Quo

We've learned a lot from the past two chapters. But you may be wondering how to face the daily challenges in this healthcare system. How can you make a real difference when the workplace is so demanding? How can you be a successful nurse while coping with stress and avoiding burnout?

The world has many types of musical instruments. There are even more music teachers, sheet music, and videos to help you learn to play. But all this means nothing to you if you don't play an instrument or if you can't read music. The same applies to your life, your health, and your goals. Many resources cover stress and burnout. But you need to know what makes you unique to find the right ones.

In this chapter, we will discuss the body's feedback mechanisms. They give you information. This info will tell you if you are at ease. Or if it's time to switch things up and get back into your groove. We will look at the bigger picture of how to start making a difference in your life right away. We will debunk common nursing myths. Then, we will create solutions for your situation.

Pause and reflect: What's your definition of a successful nurse?

Nursing success involves more than just academic credentials and perseverance alone. Success at the cost of health is short-lived.

Defining it only by external accomplishments can harm one's well-being and energy. Nurses must question their idea of success. They must redefine it to match a holistic approach to life and work.

Nursing is high-pressure. It requires long hours and big responsibilities. They can harm health, mood, and skills even without apparent stress. Eating balanced meals, staying active, and getting good sleep are essential habits. Yet, many overlook an important element: mindfulness. Without it, burnout is a real risk, even outside a clinical setting.

Success for nurses involves more than just grit. It encompasses nurturing both body and mind. Achieving a healthy work-life balance is important. Spend time on activities that bring joy, relaxation, and fulfillment outside your career. This approach keeps your passion for the job strong. It also keeps your energy balanced. It helps you burn bright, not out.

Balancing work and life is challenging, especially as responsibilities grow. But it's possible and highly rewarding. Now, my life overflows with fun, health, love, and wealth. Mastering these dynamics sheds light on why balancing work and life can be such a struggle for many of us, especially in high-pressure fields like nursing.

Giving and Receiving and Its Cycle

We are quick to help when someone needs support, going out of our way to assist them in a heartbeat. But, when we're the ones who need something, many of us struggle with asking for and accepting help. We are so hard on ourselves. Sometimes, we deny ourselves the support, love, and gifts that others offer us.

Why is that? I want to share insights from a great psychologist and my great friend, Orlando Solano, PhD. According to Solano, "Human behaviors often stem from deep-seated beliefs and past experiences. These behaviors trigger changes in our minds and bodies. They dictate how we respond to stress and challenges. Understanding these behaviors at their core lets us find patterns. This allows us to intervene early and stop burnout in its tracks.

"Why do we usually feel uncomfortable receiving? Even if it's a compliment or a kind gesture? It's because we fear that accepting help will make us vulnerable or inferior to others.

"We often avoid asking for help or support because we don't want to seem bothersome, needy, or weak. Yet, this behavior puts us in a victim mode and affects us more than we realize. We've adopted an old belief we are not worthy or deserving of receiving help.

"Several factors lead to this mindset. They include emotional damage from family, some religious teachings, our upbringing, and schools. For example, Jesus taught about living well in love, abundance, and joy. As children, we naturally receive because we believe in abundance. The message 'Ask and you shall receive' resonates with them. But, as they grow, they start getting mixed messages. For example, "Good behavior and good grades guarantee recognition." Also, "Only those who behave will receive a reward."' This teaches them to prove their worth to receive.

"A lot is often seen as greed, creating confusion and blockages. The prefrontal lobe regulates part of our conscience. It is part of our creative center and helps us make changes. The limbic system, where emotions come from experience, is also influenced. They bridge that entire discrepancy. The children's openness to receive goes down because they feel they are not good enough.

"The remaining 3-4% of the population are those of us who rebelled against this mindset. We got good at giving more love but not necessarily at receiving it. By believing that 'Hands that give are never empty,' society often conditions people not to receive, which benefits the wealthy. Poverty becomes a business. This mindset particularly affects nurses.

"Banks ensure long-term dependence through loans that span decades, affecting generations. This financial burden and emotional stress can lead to a desire for pain. Many think that enduring hardship gets you to heaven. They see having much as bad. So they assume that working hard, not being a millionaire, makes you a good person by default.

"The Franciscans are a group of Catholic religious. They focus on humility and simplicity. They rely on charity and support from others. They believe that everyone should make their own life choices. But it's wrong to impose beliefs on others. As nurses, we must find our own path to balance, embracing humility and simplicity. Like the Franciscans, we recognize that everyone's journey is unique, and true healing comes from within.

"In Japan, the approach to abundance and spirituality is healthier. After the Second World War, they changed their academic training and cultural mindset. Today, Japan blends its rich traditions with modern advancements, prospering as a first-world country while welcoming visitors. Japan strives to live in peace.

"Other first-world countries like Finland, Singapore, Switzerland, and the Netherlands provide many opportunities for people to develop. They do so even though they're considered authoritarian.

"Society flourishes when we actively support, encourage, and uplift each other. By embracing receptivity, you unlock new emotions and experiences you avoided before. (Solano, personal communication, 2024)."

This particularly affects nurses. It is scary to be open and vulnerable, fearing someone might take advantage of you. I still experience this sometimes, but it gets easier to be open to receiving, and it's rewarding and fun. Think about it. Isn't it harder to live life avoiding "what ifs"? You'd deny yourself gifts, blessings, loving memories, and opportunities out of fear.

It all starts with receiving well. Believe in yourself and your self-worth. Feel worthy of receiving. Giving is actually receiving: giving is easier. When you receive, you feel shy and hesitant but you can't become a giver without first receiving. By being a receiver, you are also giving someone the opportunity to become a giver. Their giving action is complete because of you.

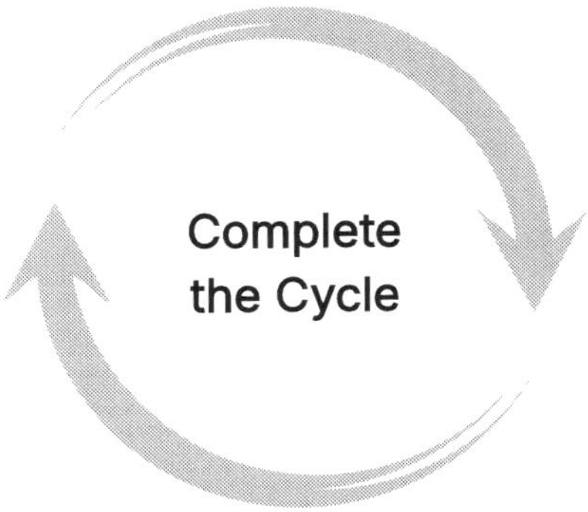

To move forward, it's important to challenge preconceived notions about success. Common burnout myths that undermine anyone's success include:

- Burnout comes from excessive hours.
- Only high-pressure jobs cause burnout.
- You can't burn out if you love your job.
- Burnout means you've failed, so it's up to you to fix it.
- Taking a vacation and pushing through will fix it.

Other myths in our profession can hinder personal growth and well-being. Raising unattainable goals and excess pressure culminates in emotional exhaustion. Debunking these myths can redefine success in nursing. It will create a more sustainable, fulfilling career. Getting rid of old ideas of success can unlock our full potential. This is true for us as individuals and as nursing professionals. It sets us up for a more balanced, satisfying career.

Debunking Myths That Could Lead to Burnout

Some myths that I will mention are not as common nowadays. Awareness surrounds them, yet it eludes many.

Perfectionism is a good trait.

As nursing students, some teachers put a lot of pressure on us. We had to know all the academic content perfectly. And, we had to apply it flawlessly during clinical rounds. There was no room for error, new perspectives, or thinking outside the box. We learned to keep busy and multitask. To follow orders without question. To work hard and put others' needs before our own. So, we assumed this path led to becoming a successful nurse.

We must excel in all our endeavors. But many factors are beyond our control or prediction. These include the patient's condition, interdepartmental issues, and insurance protocols. Regardless, many see perfectionism in nursing as normal. Some even see it as a positive trait. Some dare to say that burnout is going up because nurses aren't as tough as they used to be.

So over time, if we don't question these beliefs and we simply accept them, we start to act accordingly at work. Now, we've made it a habit. We unconsciously accept that a nurse must excel at everything while working under pressure. We end up setting exceedingly high standards for performance. Accompanied by overly critical evaluations (Stoeber, 2011).

Traits of Perfectionism

Do these traits resonate with you?

- A continuous drive to do more, be more, and prove yourself.
- A strong need for control.
- Setting impossibly high standards for yourself and others.
- Fear of failure and seeking approval from others.
- Excessive rumination and overthinking when things don't go well or when feedback is lacking
- Checking and redoing others' work.
- Inability to delegate work effectively.
- Focusing on flaws and mistakes made by others.
- Associating self-worth with career accomplishments.
- Frequent criticism of others when they don't meet your expectations.
- Excessive need for cleanliness and order.
- Presenting a perfect life to others.
- Thinking in absolutes and an inability to live with ambiguity.
- Believing that there is only one best way to achieve goals.
- Focusing on individual weaknesses versus strengths.
- Inability to be decisive without a perfect decision.
- High-stress levels during setbacks.

Some nurses are perfectionists, myself included. This trait helped us get through nursing school and excel at our jobs. What occurs when your work identity dominates your entire life?

We are bound to face hardship no matter how hard we try to prevent it. Yet, if we're not aware of this perfectionism mechanism, it can translate to other areas of our lives. Knowing when to turn off this side of you is key. These unreal expectations cause frustration, fatigue, and even shame.

People who are perfectionists usually push others away because, honestly, who wants to be with someone always running a tight ship? Do you know anyone perfect, with it all together? Exactly! No one has ever achieved this perfection. So, why are we so hard on ourselves? This is true not just as nurses but as people too.

Freeing Yourself from Perfectionism

Events from your childhood that you couldn't process led to the perfection myth. It made you believe you must be perfect to deserve love. When you spend your childhood in survival mode you seek what you know in an effort to feel safe. To create lasting change, examine your beliefs and habits. Find out why you think meeting unrealistic goals is the ultimate aim.

Practical Steps

Review all areas of your life to get started, and consider where you can set the bar lower. Focusing on done is better than perfect. What is something you can let go of or be flexible about?

Example: Is it necessary to wash the car every week? Could you invest that time and money in a rewarding experience?

1. Pick one weekly routine or habit and write down the action steps.
2. Answer these questions to ensure your plan is achievable:

- Which steps are non-negotiable each week, and which are optional?
- How can you underpromise in this action plan?
- How will you know you've accomplished the steps without feeling pressured or rushed?

Expectations are ideas you create based on your beliefs and values. When they aren't met, you suffer. The more expectations you have, the harder it is to feel happy. Write down what you do daily for a week and classify them as:

- Bringing joy or energizing you
- Done to avoid feelings of guilt or a sense of being unaccomplished.
- Done to please others.

Based on these classifications:

- How can you do more of what re-energizes you?
- What's the worst that could happen if you don't do some tasks?
- There will always be responsibilities you must do and need more of your energy and attention. So what can you change in your routine to allow more time for rest and to recharge?

Remember, our goodness doesn't come from being perfect.

Nursing students don't count

Nursing school years are unforgettable. My pet peeve is learning through fear. It tries to shatter confidence with passive-aggressive communication. This approach might have worked for some in the past, even at an elementary school level, but I don't agree with it.

I was always empathetic to others' needs, so choosing nursing as a career was a no-brainer for me. During my first semester, the joy and relief I felt in my anatomy and microbiology classes were indescribable. Studying hard wasn't the issue; it was the long commutes and treatment by teachers and hospital staff. So yeah, relationships were my issue. In my early twenties, I didn't know how to cope with rude people or bullies. Much less how to protect my peace.

Older nurses bullied us, hiding supplies and displaying rudeness. Doctors saw us as ass-wipers. Our teachers told us to keep our heads down and follow orders because that was hospital life. Ethics classes taught us what not to do but failed to address what we shouldn't tolerate.

Pause and reflect: What were your best and worst experiences as a student?

Think about how great nursing school could be if we were taught about emotion management. This includes stress, de-escalation, and active listening. Also, budgeting for new grads, and setting boundaries while interacting with tough individuals.

Addressing student mistreatment

In my first year, our clinical rotation professor only cared about the cleanliness of our shoelaces and white uniform. He didn't support us during rotations. In the 1990s in Costa Rica, you practiced all procedures with real patients in your first year. I'll never forget when a team lead (called a charge nurse back then) slapped my forearm to interrupt me. She thought I was contaminating the field while placing a Foley catheter on a female patient. Another time, we were in the ICU with a patient with a Bogota bag. As a nurse and I were bathing him, his right side sutures ruptured when we turned him towards my side of the bed. Neither of us was wearing gloves. There were not enough supplies at the hospital. She looked at me and told me to try to hold the patient's intestines in place. I was to do this until help arrived to rush the patient back to the OR. No gloves or gauze, just my bare hands. I told my professor. He blamed me for the issue, even though the nurse said we had done nothing wrong.

These experiences made me question my career choice. So I chose to play dumb, swallow my emotions, and study hard hoping things would improve after I graduated. It was a scary new world where I didn't have a voice, and that was something no one had prepared me for. My family couldn't comprehend what I was going through. Despite their best efforts to support me and be empathetic, it wasn't enough.

Reflecting on past experiences

1. Consider how these myths and experiences show up in your life. Have you faced similar situations as a student?
2. How have they changed you? How did you handle them?
3. How can you apply these insights to current situations?
4. Remember, even the toughest days shape you into the best nurse you can be.

Nurses and Doctors Are Born with Mental Toughness

A medical or nursing degree doesn't make one superhuman or immune to life's challenges. Fear, worry, and stress affect us equally. We just aren't allowed to show it openly. Yet, we often hesitate to seek help due to fear of professional repercussions. Doctors dislike seeking help because it might stain their permanent records. Nurses hesitate, too, fearing job loss or judgment from colleagues. This spreads a harmful myth—that burnout comes from personal weakness, a flaw, or poor productivity. Many view energy management, emotion regulation, and self-care as signs of weakness. It's as if tough individuals aren't supposed to behave like humans. No wonder PTSD is a serious issue among healthcare professionals. Even if the salary covers expenses and all the nice things, it often fails to bring comfort.

Moving Forward

In my last round of clinical hours, they let me choose a med/surg floor in any public hospital. So, I chose a city hospital near where I lived. When I completed my semester, the nurse manager offered me a job as an auxiliary nurse. It's a position between a CNA and an LVN that exists in Costa Rica. Not as an RN, because in Costa Rica it's hard to land a job right from the start as an RN.

At first, I was hopeful because I already knew most of the staff. But I faced bullying from nurses and got no support from management. The workload allowed none of the nurses a chance to educate patients or learn from other nurses in my case. I resigned in less than a year. I knew that things wouldn't improve, and I had almost no chance of being promoted to RN. You needed to have connections inside the system, it wasn't about how efficient you were and how much you knew. Plus, I honestly believed that more experienced nurses and charge nurses were better than me. These experiences led me to resign. I felt like the dumbest nurse in the world. I was always overthinking and dreading each shift.

Knowing when to move on without guilt is hard. This is especially true when a job was once a source of pride and identity. But sometimes, it's necessary for mental health. Think about your experiences and how they align with your values.

1. Recall one of your biggest challenges or hardest experiences as a nurse. How have they affected you?
2. If you had a guide or mentor come in and help you at that time, what would you've wanted them to do or say?

3. Could any of these experiences be the root cause of your chronic stress? As we've discussed in Chapter 2.
4. Reflect on what steps you can take to reduce this stress.
5. Can you add more self-care and realistic expectations to your role? Or is changing jobs the only way?

Remember, it's always okay to seek help and support from others.

Revamp your nursing career. Do this by shedding old wrong ideas and embracing a fresh view. It's what highlights the key skills and traits that propel nurses to success.

The Numbers Speak

It turns out I wasn't a singular case. Within two years of graduating from nursing school, 33% of nurses leave the profession. They do not return. More nurses are changing jobs. The percentage doing so keeps rising. This rise is alongside those struggling with anxiety, stress, and burnout.

A third of U.S. nurses will leave the profession post-COVID-19, while 36% plan to stay but switch workplaces. A survey of over 18,000 nurses demands change; 69% want higher salaries, and 63% need a safer work environment to reduce stress.

The survey was from NCBI. It was between January and March 2021. It found that about two-thirds of nurses (65.6%) reported high job burnout. Another NCBI survey of 431 nurses showed 50.8% had stress, 74% had anxiety, and 70.8% had depression. 79.1% experienced at least one of these conditions.

We have little information about workplace stress and negative emotions among nurses. But these surveys show that ongoing job stress can harm mental health. It can also harm patient care.

Today, after a global pandemic, 62% of U.S. nurses report symptoms related to burnout. This is from a recent national survey by the American Nurses Association.

Employers should focus on supporting and keeping nurses. By creating a safe workplace, valuing mental health, and promoting seeking help when needed. Yet, many corporate managers overlook the concerns raised by front-line and mid-level managers. I'll explain this further shortly.

Change jobs and you'll be fine.

The approach to work is different now compared to 15-20 years ago. Nowadays, nurses seek advice even from social media groups. Informing themselves on transitioning from bedside roles to administrative or specialized positions. When I was a bedside nurse, I was clueless about these options. The only solution I knew about was working at another hospital. I had no idea about the opportunities available beyond bedside nursing.

Some make the shift and fall in love with the profession again. Others realize that no place is good enough due to the current healthcare challenges. Those who move to the corporate world often find working three days a week more manageable than the traditional 8-5, five days a week. However, nurses in care manager or Utilization Management roles sometimes face heavy workloads. Paired with micromanagement and extensive documentation tasks that can extend beyond paid hours. It's also hard on the mind and body to sit for long hours at a desk with few breaks.

Identify your ideal job by understanding yourself first. Consider your personality, skills, and needs. Your values and life stage also play a significant role. Once you know who you are and what matters to you, you'll find the job that fits.

My Journey

When I moved to Austin, Texas, from Costa Rica in 2000, I experienced a never-before joy of being a nurse. The level of respect that nurses had in the USA blew me away. For the first time, most doctors listened. Fellow nurses and CNAs willingly helped when the workload was insane.

Yet, as the years went by while working in the Telemetry and IMC unit, I started to notice a pattern. The better you are and the more you work, the more responsibilities you get. I often worked with the most difficult patients and would stay late to finish my charting. When I talked to my nurse manager about it, she said she appreciated my ability to handle stress in a busy setting, which is why I got those patients. But I didn't see a raise in my pay despite the acknowledgment.

After working briefly as a relief charge nurse, I was offered the charge nurse position for the weekends, but I respectfully declined. I wasn't sure of my abilities then. A doctor of Electrophysiology recognized my great judgment and proactive approach. Then, his team offered me a transfer to the EP lab. I was thrilled, hoping it would reduce my stress and exhaustion. Boy, was I wrong! The workload in the EP lab was heavy in a different way. Working 16-hour days, five days a week, took a toll on my marriage and left me burnt out.

I adopted many unhealthy coping mechanisms. These included junk food, alcohol, and sleeping pills. I was on diuretics for fluid retention. And I was on appetite suppressants for weight gain. I gained weight from long work hours, lack of exercise, and poor eating habits. I was only in my mid-20s and felt 80 years old! My manager suggested transferring to the Cath Lab for fewer hours. But being on call created a whole new level of anxiety for me.

Developing a minor arrhythmia terrified me. I hungered for escape but lacked a clear direction. My husband was in medical school, so we depended on my income.

Reflection

Changing jobs isn't always the solution. It's essential to consider the factors contributing to your decision to leave. All jobs have pros and cons. But it might be the amount of stress you face. Or it might be a mix of job duties and stress. Finding purpose again will give you the clarity to make good choices.

1. How does this myth show up in your life?
2. Have you considered changing jobs? Why?
3. Write down the pros and cons of your current role. What would your ideal job look like?
4. How can you get clarity about your next steps?
5. Have you considered improving your current work environment first? What resources would you need?
6. If you've already changed jobs, what was the outcome? Did it solve your issues? What actions would you change in retrospect?
7. **Final Thought:** Sometimes, the grass is greener where you water it.

I'm Just a Nurse

Some nurses want to explore new roles but feel nervous. They fear taking on new tasks, changing their self-image, making errors, and facing the unknown. Colleagues and traditional ideas about moving away from direct patient care can add pressure. As a result, some nurses hesitate to act, lacking the guidance and encouragement needed to switch careers.

I started as a care manager for wellness programs. Then, I became the first and only board-certified Nurse Coach for a digital health giant. Later, I worked as a clinical coach. I co-created the entire program's SOPs. I also worked as a copywriter, personal assistant, corporate consultant, and marketing strategist. I was also the lead clinical research nurse for groundbreaking discoveries.

The phrase *I'm just a nurse* grossly understates the remarkable work we do daily. I've helped many nurses transition careers. They'll attest that we're not just capable - we're essential.

Nurses have a unique blend of skills and training they can apply in various settings. We excel at communication. We can handle pressure. We are good at multitasking, critical thinking, and quick decision-making. These skills are valuable in fast-paced environments. Our compassion and empathy help us excel in customer service and human resources. We also bring strengths to administrative and managerial roles. These include paying attention to detail and being organized.

When I left the hospital as a single mom, I looked into work-from-home options. I also considered hiring a nanny to spend more time with my daughter. As I read the job requirements, I cringed. I would say, "But I'm just a nurse. I don't have those skills or corporate experience." Imposter syndrome hit hard.

I felt uncomfortable applying for jobs outside my experience. But to my surprise, most employers I applied to interviewed me. I thought they would ignore me. My first job required me to work closely with other case managers and Utilization Management nurses. I didn't feel as competent or intelligent as my co-workers. Any minor mistake or feedback, even if it was positive, from my manager made me overthink everything! I would think, "They're gonna discover the truth about me. I'm not good enough for this role." Anxiety still ruled most of my life. I was out of my comfort zone. But my daughter needed me to step up, and she gave me the courage to do so. Love always makes the hard things possible.

I felt pressure to perform at my best all the time. It was no joke. When I didn't, I felt incompetent. I became a course junkie to calm my fears and anxiety. Any course or certification that was available, I immediately signed up for it.

Years went by, and despite feeling like an imposter, I'd succeeded in these roles. Perfectionism[32] can contribute to imposter syndrome. It was all in my head!

Yet, it was so hard to convince myself of this. I didn't know any mindfulness practices; I used to think that going for a walk, yoga, and tai chi was a waste of time. All that unnecessary worry about not fitting in, combined with the silent, lingering stress of not managing my energy levels, deeply affected me. It ultimately led to my second burnout, even outside a clinical setting, and my diagnosis with an autoimmune disease.

1. How does this myth show up in your life?
2. What has your journey been like? Have you ever felt less capable than another professional?
3. Has fear held you back from taking the first step toward your new job? Remember, it's unfamiliarity that causes fear, not incapability.
4. Changing this deep belief won't happen overnight. But the following suggestions can help you cope with imposter syndrome.
    - Reflect on your concrete achievements and how far you've come.

- Remind yourself that it's scary because it's unfamiliar, not because you're incapable. Being nervous and anxious is a normal part of the process. Give yourself grace as you grow.
- Share your feelings with a loved one. Ideally, outside of the setting in which you feel like an impostor.

5. Seek a mentor who has charted a similar path.
6. Accept mistakes as a natural part of early attempts at new experiences. Challenges can lead to mistakes but also to growth. Mistakes are an unavoidable part of life, and you shouldn't fear them.

But through it all, I learned the most important nursing skill nobody ever taught us: how to live with a mistake. So, remember, failure isn't the enemy—it's your ticket to growth and success. I explore this essential topic in more depth in Chapter 6. Feeling like an imposter means you need more practice becoming the person you aspire to be. Comparison can either help or hurt, depending on how you see it. Keep going, keep refining, and keep calibrating to that next level. Eventually, that role you're dreaming of will feel like second nature—a hand-in-glove fit.

Nurses will never be wealthy

Between student loan debt and other financial obligations, money management is stressful. This is especially true for overworked nurses on the brink of burnout. Financial stress affects millions daily. It is a leading cause of mental health issues in the U.S. However, nurses are especially vulnerable. Since they invest little time in financial literacy.

Your health and time are your most valuable assets. Some nurses trade time for more money. They do this without questioning the toll on their minds and bodies. Even if they are aware, they still agree because they don't believe there is another way to make more money. I get it; for many years, I struggled to pay the bills and afford groceries. Trying to make ends meet each month, despite working hard and taking on extra shifts, was stressful. It bought me an express pass to the burnout train. Even if you invest time daily in self-care and mindfulness, it's depleting.

I used to believe that my money problems would fix themselves. I thought some event or person would intervene somehow. I was stuck in a mindset that shifted the blame, refusing to own up to my choices and actions. The moment I took full responsibility and stopped waiting for external fixes. When I channeled my energy and attention into my finances, I had significant growth.

So, what can you do to stay afloat and improve your financial situation?

You can achieve financial peace with proper guidance and support. Financial wellness is a thing. Ken Honda mentored me, and I'm lucky to have had that opportunity. He is an international expert in true wealth and financial freedom. He advises that money is energy. So, focus on managing your feelings about it. Practice gratitude for what you have. And seek ways to improve your money skills and situation without stress or fear.

A healthier relationship with money can reduce debt and financial stress. Additionally, generating passive income with your current earnings is possible. You can save this extra income for retirement, emergencies, or higher education. Or my favorite- for traveling!

We have a huge advantage as nurses to create both passive and active income. Active income includes per diem shifts, overtime, travel nursing, consulting, and entrepreneurship. Passive income can come from royalties from writing and publishing online courses and webinars, and investments in real estate or the stock market.

Building a foundation you can stand on for the rest of your life is not just about money. It's about being open to new perspectives.

Make peace with your money and recognize that your nursing degree is more than enough. Don't feel pressured to get another degree or certification to prove your worth. First, feel proud, satisfied, and accomplished. Then, think about academic or career progress because you choose to, not because you must.

Financial Self-Assessment

1. What have been your major struggles regarding money?
2. What have you tried so far?
3. One common mistake is trying to fix your financial issues by making more money. First, you must look at your current expenses and lower them. Track your budget weekly or monthly. Cut out the unnecessary expenses, such as unused apps, memberships, and TV cable. Plan your grocery shopping weekly and look for discounts or bulk products.
4. Which forms of income interest you the most? Pick one and start researching how to get started.
5. Ask for advice and support from people you trust with a stable financial situation. Fast and easy financial freedom proposals rarely end well.
6. Follow nurses doing similar things and learn from them. Or hire a coach to learn how to use your expertise and time to increase your income. Many nurses like me are breaking barriers every day. We break stereotypes, support communities in need, and achieve financial independence. Stay curious and open-minded, and explore the right paths that suit your personality.

7. Pick up extra shifts or side hustles only after you are clear on your spending patterns. Many of us, including myself in the past, often spend more money than we intend. We often choose to spend money on things that are not essential but that are enjoyable. For example, choosing fancier homes. Picking up the latest cell phone models. Going for luxury cars instead of cheaper ones. And buying branded clothing.

Financial freedom for nurses is within reach—take the first step! Remember, if you don't fix the root cause, the more you make, the more you will spend.

Have you ever thought about why many healthcare chains do not give nurses big raises or bonuses?

Understanding these industry dynamics can give you insight into the financial challenges nurses face and why it's crucial to take control of your finances. Focus on improving your financial situation by starting small and being consistent. Your financial peace is within reach with the right tools and mindset.

Understanding the Journey

Nurses' main issues are staffing ratios and low pay. These have lasted for over 100 years. Nurses had direct economic ties to patients in the late 1800s and early 1900s. They operated as independent businesses. However, by the 1930s, nurses became hospital employees, losing their economic independence. Hospital leaders sought to hide nurses' value. They did this by adding nursing costs to room rates. This practice continues today.

Nurses remain the only healthcare professionals not billed as a service. The nursing profession faces repeated cost-cutting, affecting patient safety and healthcare. It's time to reconsider how we organize nursing care. We need to explore new payment models and address the business side of nursing. This is how we can build a healthcare system that focuses on preventive care and cure.

Final Thoughts

Everyone wants to succeed. There is little difference between wins and failures; both are necessary parts of success. As we go through life, we enjoy the victories but grow through the struggles. We need those struggles to grow. So, take your rest as seriously as your work. Achieving a healthy work-life balance and adding self-improvement habits to your daily routine will create new experiences and opportunities, energizing you with fresh emotions.

Your journey is unique. Don't let others' opinions stop you from finding your path. You can be, do, and have more! Do the best you can, keep growing, and you will succeed.

Testimony: A Nurse's Perspective

As we explore the nuances of stress and its impacts, hearing from others who have faced similar challenges can be enlightening. Below is a testimony from fellow nurses, sharing their experience with stress, the myths, and how they navigated through it.

- **Nursing Resiliency: 36 years at the bedside (and beyond!)-** *By Ankhasanamen Sow, RN,MSN,HMCT. A bedside Labor and Delivery RN for 36 years*

The career of nursing is not a sprint, it's a marathon. As novice nurses enter this marathon, full of energy and ideas, goals and aspirations, they may experience the track they are starting on as rocky, and then smooths out for as they enter into experience... or vice versa (for a beautiful examination of this, see Patricia Brenner's book *From Novice to Expert: Excellence and Power in Clinical Nursing Practice*).

During the marathon, one should not miss the opportunity to stop and catch one's breath, take the literal and proverbial sips of water and avoid the temptation to compare one's self to the other runners...the marathon is yours and yours alone.

I knew early on that my goal was never to stay at one facility for 30 years and then retire with a comfy pension or fat 401k. My goal was to experience nursing beyond my hometown, home state, and, ultimately, my country. What I didn't realize until later in my career was that would be my ticket to avoiding burnout.

By taking side jobs at other hospitals, I benefited in several ways. I discovered that things are done differently from facility to facility, even in the same town. As I took occasional travel jobs outside of my state, I learned there were regional differences. This provided me with new and often powerful ways of providing care I collected into my little black bag of patient care tricks of the trade.

Another benefit I gained was that having to apply for new jobs and the required tests, getting to find my way around a new unit and hospital, learning a new charting system, meeting new staff members and doctors (and their names), switching from working with residents vs. private doctors, etc., all helped in keeping me on top of my game. By consistently stepping into the unknown kept me in a state of heightened awareness...no sleepwalking in the world of the familiar and sometimes worn-out neuro pathways that can destroy critical thinking over time. These new experiences sometimes allowed for a breath of fresh air... or occasionally, made me appreciate my home-base hospital even more!

All these travel side gigs were possible because early on and for the vast majority of my 36+ years at the bedside, I have maintained per- diem jobs as a home base. Being a per-diem nurse has given me the endurance for this longevity in an increasingly challenging career.

Whenever I find myself in my personal tells of upcoming burnout, I can take as long a break as I need while still satisfying my per-diem minimum requirements. I made more by the hour than my regular staff position, so I could afford to buy my own health insurance, save for time off vacations that I didn't need to compete for, and keep myself fresh and in the zone by working in new environments.

If there is a downside, for some it may be the perceived lack of security for retirement. My perception is that consistently stepping into the unknown, surviving, and thriving in each new experience has given me the confidence to now move away from the bedside into a new unknown: starting a business as a nurse entrepreneur. I am familiar with the discomfort of being a novice and being in the unknown. My method of escaping burnout by being a career per-diem nurse may not be a choice for many. However, it can be an option when burnout arrives: it can be a temporary career break... do it for a time, survey the career field and then take a staff position again. For me, it's been my life: while I kept my Labor and Delivery per diem, I did travel positions across the country and to the U.S. Virgin Islands; worked for 2 years as a middle-school nurse who volunteered in Haiti. I even left my per-diem job and spent 3 years working with MSF/ Doctors Without Borders in West and East Africa and Haiti. All these experiences have made me a more well-rounded person and a better nurse, keeping my career fresh. This has given me a resiliency that has supported me in 36 years of being able to work at the bedside; not as an endurance through burnout, but rather on my terms. I get to choose to win this marathon with ease and flow, healthy and excited for what's next!

Back to the Bedside - *By Brenna Blanchette, RN.*

I worked hard to get into nursing school, feeling a profound sense of honor, duty, and responsibility to provide excellent care and stay knowledgeable, current, and relevant in my standards of practice. I entered nursing with a love for science and to be part of people's healing journeys, to help them heal, see them change for the better, and help them in any way I could.

One of the parts I loved most was checking my patients' lab work and seeing their improvements, such as a decrease in WBC count or improved kidney function. I would arrive early for my shift and look up my patients. Results Review was something I always looked forward to, where I could see the tangible outcomes of acute care efforts through patients' imaging, labs, and pathology reports.

However, over the years, I began to question the true impact of my work. I felt I was part of a system that conditioned patients to believe they had little autonomy or control over their bodies and limited influence over their outcomes. Patients often left the hospital on multiple new medications, told they would need them for a lifetime, terrified of missing a PT appointment without understanding they could also perform certain exercises independently beyond their prescribed sessions. Some patients believed a missed appointment or a missed pill would define their outcome.

Working at two of the top hospitals in the country, always striving for excellence, innovation, and progression in patient care, I had two profound experiences that shifted the course of my nursing career. At a top-ranked hospital, I followed a diabetic educator as they provided a newly diagnosed type 2 diabetic patient with an hour of one-on-one teaching before discharge. Despite the thorough education on using a glucometer, insulin dosing, managing sharps containers, insulin storage, and various other supplies, I was struck by the lack of emphasis on lifestyle modifications, diet, and exercise. I was told, "Medicare only reimburses for an approved educational curriculum," which left me speechless.

At another hospital, amid the COVID-19 pandemic in 2022, I saw two doctors arguing about the hospital's COVID-19 policies in the patient's room, in front of the patient and me. This lack of consistent, evidence-based practice pushed me to reconsider my path, leading me to take a break from the hospital.

I chose to clean houses, finding peace and fulfillment in nurturing people through their environments. I did not have the stress of nursing in the acute care hospital setting, and financial compensation was also greater than what 14 years of acute care nursing yielded.

Returning to acute care with a new perspective has been a transformative experience. My patients now engage in breath work, create "I am" statements, and understand they are the most influential factor in their outcomes. I've learned to maintain a balance, no longer saying yes to direct text messages from managers and supervisors to pick up shifts (28 out of 30 days of the month had inadequate nursing staff) out of guilt or a desire to help, knowing it's not sustainable.

What was once a pattern of convergent focus and day-to-day survival has evolved into a divergent focus of living and working in alignment with what I know to be true for long-term career sustainability. I am forever grateful for the opportunity and gift of nursing. "Burn Bright, Not Out" beautifully encapsulates this evolution, offering invaluable insights for anyone in the nursing profession who desires to stay in their heart and in the nursing profession.

From Bedside Warrior to Advocate for Change: My Journey in Nursing, searching for a healthier path. - *By Patricia Daiker RN, NC-BC. VP of Clinical Operations, Product Manager, Holistic Nurse, and Owner of Better Diabetes Life.*

I began my nursing career at age 20, and the norm was to care for everyone but yourself. In those days, we had to give our seats to doctors when they entered the nurses' station and empty their ashtrays! Luckily, over the years, that paradigm has shifted, but nurses are still expected to put forth far more than is healthy - emotionally or physically.

From floor nursing to ICU to a Level 1 Trauma center, I worked long hours, never got enough sleep, and food and bathroom breaks were not a priority if anyone else needed anything. I miss the days of at least having enough staffing to give back rubs - yes, we did that! I felt I knew my patients and was comfortable coordinating the care among all the specialists. But as payment plans shifted with DRGs and new managed care initiatives, more and more was expected with less and less. I have been through periods of hiring freezes, elimination of patient care assistants, and too much mandatory overtime to count.

During my time in the ER, we were considered a self-contained unit and didn't pull from staffing in other parts of the hospital, or use any agency. Our staff was all we had, so it wasn't unusual to get an extra 12-hour shift added to your schedule. It was four 12-hour night shifts, 1 day off, then another four shifts to finally get 5 days off. It was brutal, and I was exhausted most of the time. But we became a family that supported each other; the docs, the nurses, and the techs bonded like a military family. And with what we saw daily, war zone was not a bad analogy. That is how we made it through. We trusted each other. We told bawdy jokes and pretended we were fine when we did CPR on a baby and then had to cater to an affluent client who wanted more narcotics. No one mentioned mental health or offered counseling when a police officer was shot, but we saw the effects. I made my decision to leave the bedside when I looked at the impact 20 years of ER had on some of my co-workers. I remember calling them crispy because they were so burnt out. I knew that would be me if I didn't make changes.

Ironically enough, life helped me make that decision. Although I can't prove it, I know there is a correlation between the workload I endured and a diagnosis of type 1 diabetes at age 26 while working in the ER. It was probably triggered by some viral infection from a patient I had cared for, but I also know my immune system was shot from chronic stress, overwhelm, and exhaustion. It was a lethal combo. I stayed in the ER, doing bedside care for several more years, but looked for gentler, kinder ways to earn my dollars and take care of my health. Eventually, I left the bedside to work for an ER software vendor. It was a different kind of stress for sure, but I had more control of my environment, I felt my contributions were recognized, and I used my years at the bedside to help those still in the ER. It gave me my life back, and I missed the ER, but my sanity was worth it.

As I reflect, we were all burned out, but there were no words for it back then. We did what we did and assumed it was normal. It saddens me that today nurses continue to be asked to provide more than 60 minutes of care in each hour they work. They remain the important bridge between a dangerous healthcare system that is too focused on metrics, outcomes, and patient satisfaction scores and the vulnerable patients with no other choice. They must know when to call a provider, when to stop, when to go, when to give the drug, when to hold the drug, and when a physical symptom is significant. They are the glue that holds the system together...for now. But everyone has their limits. It's time to reinvent this broken system.

04 The Human Side of Healthcare Leadership

I'm tackling stress and burnout head-on because they're deeply personal. I know social pressure plays a significant role in causing them, so I want to bring up an important subject that's close to my heart. It's about how nurses see their healthcare leaders. And what we can do to make our jobs easier.

Every single human experiences the same range of emotions. The difference is in how these emotions manifest. Leaders and managers also cherish the love, joy, and fulfillment you experience, and they also grapple with fear, worry, and guilt. Being a leader in this healthcare system is a challenging and often misunderstood road. When team leaders, front-line staff, and mid-line managers lack support from their superiors, dealing with stress and recovering from burnout can be hard. This often shows up in their behavior, actions, and communication efforts.

We must recognize that stress, division, and uncertainty surround us, but we hold the power to create inner calm and composure. By listening to one another, we can break down barriers and make everyone feel heard, understood, and valued.

I want to share with you powerful interviews with two directors of major healthcare chains in the USA. They will help you understand what they endure daily and why changing this healthcare system is so hard.

Interview with Liz, Semi-Retired Director

Q: Please share what your journey has been like over the past thirty years.

Liz: I've been a nurse for 30 years, working at six hospitals in Texas. I've seen burnout at many levels among nurses and leaders, and I've lived through it personally. So I'm passionate about this topic.

My background is in critical care, and I worked for 14 years at the bedside. Even in my first years, I led committees and was a representative in many meetings. Even as a new grad, people considered me a natural leader. I earned a master's in business administration. I worked as a House Supervisor and Education Coordinator. My first manager role was in Pediatrics. A specialty in which I had no patient care experience, but it was fun and easy to cut your deed as a manager. Pediatrics makes a lot of money. So, staffing was never a problem. Turnover was not a problem. The schedule and budget were not problems either. I joined a formal mentorship program while in this role. I worked for 23 years at a Magnet Hospital that offered it. My mentor was a director. A chief nursing officer guided me to a director role at a community hospital, where I served for five years before I burned out.

Turns out that a manager role is harder than a director role. Staffing and meeting productivity requirements are tough to meet. I was living through the challenges. It was the first time that I realized both and that it's different from any other industry. Only in healthcare, you are responsible for everything that happens within your department. The scope is wide. You're tasked with things like productivity, turnover, and quality. You're also responsible for employee engagement.

Struggling to disconnect from work and being held accountable 24/7. I would check my emails right before bed or as soon as I was awake to know what happened overnight from the house supervisor. That's how it was for 5 years at this small medical center.

My scope was larger at this smaller hospital than when I worked at the bigger ones. To show you, during the COVID pandemic, I was the ICU, IMC, and Telemetry director. Comprising 8 beds respectively and 64 floor beds. To support my team from 2013 to 2018, I worked 12 hours a day, 7 days a week nonstop. Sometimes I had only two nurses scheduled to take care of 8 ICU patients. There was no crisis response support, no travel nurses, no aid. The workload was insane. During those years, I learned a valuable lesson in hindsight. I should have stood up more and demanded a bigger pool of nurses and that non-clinical nurses, such as educators and quality care personnel, come in to help us when we were short-staffed.

In 2012-2014, the hospitals were struggling to make a profit. So, there was increased accountability on directors from the accountant consultants who came in and gave their productivity targets to meet. It was a stressful organizational focus. They changed the Medicare rules so hospitals are more accountable for the patient experience but only focused on money and reimbursement.

Medicare and Medicaid standardized the patient experience questionnaire for inpatients. It asked about the call light responsiveness and side effects of meds among other things.

There were five questions in each category. So all hospitals started to focus on the same things. Because of this, to help hospital organizations, along came consultants from the Studer Group. They trained us to script answers correctly while we did the patient rounding. We learned how to talk to them so they can answer the questions correctly. Targeting their experience. The performance on the survey meant more dollars. It's all about money, money, money!

This productivity and patient experience focus both became very micromanaged by the organization. The stress and focus on us directors to meet those metrics was elevated. In my leadership, I kept my eyes on the right things while hoping that the organization would leave me alone. My two core tenets were:

1. Best possible patient care.
2. Create a work environment that is the healthiest possible for my employees.

I believed that if I were a good leader and did things my way, it would all work out. Good will and good smart leadership acumen. But that's not how organizations work.

My everyday life became very, and I mean very micromanaged. Meetings took up my entire day. There weren't enough hours in the day to get it all done. I was given unrealistic expectations or directives that weren't achievable. The productivity target for the ICU was calculated by some 25-year-old consultant, who had been paid to come and tell the top-level managers this. But when I started doing the math, looking at the census and daily turnover, I realized that the target for my unit was not even mathematically achievable. It wasn't humanly possible. Questioning that just led to a belief that it was work that I couldn't tolerate, that I was the issue, so eventually, I quit.

I quit without a plan, a crossroads in terms of my career at age 40 in 2016. I was off for 7 months, with no structure or time management. I was lucky to have other sources of income. So going back to work due to money was not a pressure. After a few months of reflection, I realized that I loved my job and that I was a good director. I loved the scope of responsibility, helping lead a team, and understanding and loving the new nurses. So, I got back on the horse but decided to switch companies to see if there would be any difference. In my state there were only two healthcare chains. Turns out they had the same scope of services and size but they only hired internally. I applied to several jobs as a Director but didn't get them. So, after 10 years, I decided to become a staff nurse again. It was scary! Going from working as an ICU nurse to an ER nurse. I applied, and within 24 hours, I got a job. I went up to the CNO and introduced myself during orientation. She told me to set up an appointment after a month of working for them. So, I was an ER nurse for a few months and then became the ICU director in 2017. I was in charge of the ICU, IMC, telemetry unit, and chaplain services from 2017 to 2019. It was a nice, fun job. I could use my skill set with my people. Hire and take good care of the new grads. Promoting a healthy work environment with parties for all staff members.

Then, from March 2020 to 2022, we had four waves of Covid patients a few months apart. It was overwhelming due to the staffing challenges, high acuity, and a lot of patient deaths. We had over 300 deaths in the ICU. We had FEMA nurses six days a week, and we took over the Cath lab to have more ICU beds.

I became very consumed with epidemiology and following ventilator rates. To have some sense of control—in retrospect. I read the articles in The Atlantic and provided daily updates in May and June 2020 to my team.

It was hard to keep up because management kept changing policies quickly because nobody knew what was going on. One day, they would order us to intubate early, then the next day, they would tell us not to intubate. So, I created a private FB page for 100 nurses to share updates in less time. Despite my best efforts, it was just too much on me, so I quit in May 2022. I was a Director for 10 years and quit for the second time. All the fun, pride, and joy got erased with this pandemic. Corporate got very controlling and micromanaged every aspect of the hospital. There was no autonomy left for the Directors or Operators at individual hospitals. We had daily calls with all the hospital leaders to unify strategies in every single way. Squeezed out of the joy of my role. All the fun was gone. This, paired with the 2 years of the complete inability to unplug, was what led me to quit.

I remember that August 2021 was the last wave and the worst spike. I was on a two-week vacation and couldn't rest or relax. While away, I was still checking in daily with my staff. I dreaded going back because I knew exactly what I would walk into from the previous COVID waves. So, that fall was when I decided I couldn't do this anymore. It took a big toll on me, and my mental health was suffering. So, I stayed until that winter to be there for my team.

My life is good now. The last 2 years have been great, but I had to grieve, and I guess I still am (as she's crying). Leaving a job that I loved and that I was good at. Some of it was the pandemic and no one's fault, but some of it was corporate greed. Actually, most of the fault falls on corporate greed. The hospitals, as publicly traded companies, are accountable to their shareholders first. The CEOs are mandated to make the most profit possible. It is their sole goal. So, they squeeze employees in every possible way to maximize profit.

One glaring example of this is the staffing challenges brought on by the COVID pandemic. Waves of great nurses resigned for obvious reasons like the risk of COVID, the overwhelming acuity, and death rates. As a result, staffing ratios changed out of necessity, like the IMC that used to have a 4:1 patient-to-nurse ratio pre-pandemic. Now, it's a 5-6-7:1 patient-to-nurse ratio. Once the pandemic ended, we should have gone back to normal, but those ratios stayed the same. And that's just wrong, anytime, taking care of 7 patients during the day or night shift. It's all just greed and profit.

I'm angry about that, but I also recognized that I no longer wanted to be the face, the messenger because that's what directors do. They're the interface between corporate (the operators and top-level leaders) and the frontline staff. Directors are in the middle.

I didn't want to give the message that 7:1 was the new normal. Another scenario was that the standard number of ICU nurses per shift was 16. With the pandemic, it went up to 22-23. Post-pandemic, we were lucky to have 12. So 12 was the new 16. That was the joke among the supervisors. 12 is the new 16...

It all falls on the back of the frontline nurses. The workload is the same, and they want to take excellent care of their patients but simply can't.

Q: As a director, did they offer any support to you? Did you ask for resources and receive them?

Liz: Since my employer is the largest American for-profit operator of healthcare facilities, they would send flyers in the mail to offer doctors and PCP services on demand. I don't know if it was just lip service or if it was real. I have 2 family members who are psychiatrists, so I spoke with them and never used the services from my employer. I also relied a lot on my friends; we even created a peer support group. But I feel like my employer tried. My team never mentioned if they used them, it was kinda like a taboo...

As a director, what message would you share with the frontline nurses?

Liz: Now I'm a staff nurse again, working in the Cath lab, so the burdens and challenges I now face as a staff nurse are different. But I realized that if I'm a squeaky wheel, my challenges will get addressed. But as a Director, if it's related to productivity or a cheaper supply option, then it's simply not gonna happen. When it's about dollars and costs to the Corporation, nothing changes.

So now that I'm a front-line nurse, I make daily calculations, and I ask myself:

- Is it worth it for me to be here? Because I can go and get another job tomorrow.
- Is my experience here worth it? Regarding the frustration, the workload, the stress, the physical toll.
- Is the cost worth it?

So far, yes.

Because I'm making a difference, one patient at a time. I can reassure them, keep them safe, and get genuine appreciation for them. Even though the physical toll is a lot. We usually have 10 cases per day. Some days, we have help, but not always. At 54, it feels like a workout, and I enjoy it, but other times, I don't want to hurt my back.

Frontline nurses need to keep asking themselves and make that calculation individually because some things can improve and get fixed if you're a squeaky wheel. But the big picture of profit motivation and staffing ratios that benefit the organization and not the nurse isn't gonna change anytime soon. Or even if you're working for a for-profit company, that's just the way it is. The only thing you can do about it is be empowered to do what you can do in your world.

That means treating your coworkers well and being supportive as a team. As a staff nurse, you have to focus on the things you have control over, which is a small environment, like your interactions with your patients and coworkers or other professionals. I know it's not the most positive message, and you might feel powerless to make a big change, but after thirty years as a nurse in multiple roles, I've accepted that a staff nurse has little power.

Now that being said, we have the power to decide when we're gonna cut corners. Safety or time-wise, when you're pressured to provide patient care. You have the power in terms of how you respond to pressures. I'm not gonna run down the hall to get more patients faster. You have the agency to do it your way. And if we, collectively, have agency, a unified collective voice, then we also have unified collective power.

I am pro-union now, so they can negotiate on behalf of employees. It makes sense now. We need more bargaining power for mandated ratios like California has now.

Q: Do you have any advice for other leaders?

Liz: Yes. Hold on to your integrity. If you're asked to be the messenger or to do some Corporate Mandate thing you know is not right, say no. You need to have integrity and courage. I know that it is hard because people need their jobs.

Unfortunately, what I felt I needed to do to preserve my mental health and my sanity ultimately was to maintain a healthy work-life balance and not work myself to the grave. But I wasn't able to pull it off. So I'm not the right person to advise on this. I wasn't able to pick and choose. Because you see, as a Director, what you are asked to do is impossible timewise. It's kinda like the productivity example I gave before. The target is not mathematically achievable. The same is true for us time-wise. You can only focus on 4-5 big-ticket things in your job. But when you're given 20, you have to pick and choose. But you're not given the authority to pick and choose for yourself, so you decide which checkbox to mark. Because I'm not really gonna do the work. All they want to see is the list marked off and which task you're devoting your attention to. So it was hard for me to decide, almost impossible to let things go and fall to the side. For big for-profit companies, like this one, what gets their attention is what breaks. If something fails or breaks. As a leader, you pick what you're gonna let fail or break. But it's hard to let it break or fail. It takes a lot of courage, and if you're like me, OCD and highly accountable, aiming to achieve tasks with integrity, it's hard. Add to that the hospital corporate structure, where they tell you to make this happen and do it in this way. It's prescriptive. You're told to do X, Y, and Z, knowing that it's not gonna make a difference in the outcome. Being forced daily on every shift, that's also a crazy-making tension. Because you still do it even though it has nothing to do with the outcome. Everybody knew this. Just check the box because somebody at a high corporate level came up with it. It was intangible and intolerable for me.

Interview with Mike, Director and Senior Manager

Q: What do you think are the major sources of burnout for nurses and managers?

Mike: When you're an employee, you have some mental commitment. In my case, it was related to my unit suffering, so I needed to go in and help. Leaders tried to go above and beyond to try and help. This was accentuated during the pandemic. But it's a similar effect to what nurses nowadays are experiencing with non-nursing duties...

Day shift nurses are on the phone with the Nutrition department for five minutes to get ketchup because nobody answers the phone or she must go to the fridge to get it. It all adds up. All those non-necessary acute care duties add up. Or the wound wrap for the patient wasn't available, but it's 6 pm or it's the weekend, so no one is available at the supplies department. So she must call the house supervisor and wait for it. So the nurse spends, on average, 2-3 hours looking for supplies or other non-clinical duties, 4-5 hours in documentation, plus their nursing duties. The lack of support and resources is affecting them. There must be a way to improve supply chain support and documentation software policies. Logistics and inventory alone aren't enough.

Leaders must deal with meeting burnout. Most of their time is spent in KPI meetings, board care, finance, and morning huddles. Sometimes, they are driving or at lunch while also attending meetings. Some have suffered DVTs and other health issues due to long sitting hours. Some tried to ask for a standing desk and got denied or had to endure a long approval process. Corporate leaders don't understand that it's better to invest in a $2,000 standing desk for their employees rather than having the employee deal with the medical costs plus absence days from work due to a DVT.

So yes, nurse leaders are also suffering. They constantly receive calls after 7 pm or on weekends and must respond to them even if they have worked over 40 hours that week.

Q: What would you say is the biggest contributing factor?

Mike: Open communication is often misunderstood as negativity, but I'm simply advocating for my team. My primary responsibility is to the people below or beneath my downline—those who trust me or report to me. Making the hospital or organization look and do better is great, but at the end of the day, if I'm not providing or supporting my team, there's no meaning to my work.

Because they're the ones taking care of those patients. My job is to take care of them. So yes, open communication is beneficial with those ancillary departments that might be helpful. That's why it's important to be firm, not rude.

Leaders must be visible and stand up for their teams. It's a big responsibility. Be observant, go around. Ask questions and do meaningful actions. Follow up on the feedback that you received from your team. Keep them in the loop. Explain how you took care of that concern they had. If you couldn't or didn't, be honest about it. Share what you tried to do about it. Be kind, consistent, fair, and be the light. Be a source of light; strive to bring positivity, hope, and inspiration to those around you.

Q: How many leaders are holistic, proactive, and down-to-earth?

Mike: It's a vicious cycle because you need time to think and plan for things. But if the projects and tasks just pile up, you get overwhelmed. They just can't put it aside and see the clear skies. So, yes, talk to your supervisor about your workload or your support person. A work buddy. Even at a CNO level, you need someone to vent, compare approaches, bounce ideas, and set priorities.

In the past, any new deadlines would take a month to a week or one week to one day to get done. But today, employers demand more and faster. They have no patience.

Leaders also need to change these perspectives and say: "Okay, it's not time now. I will look into that when I can. Set boundaries. Take care of what you can right away. If it's quick and easy, do it right away. So that your list of tasks is smaller each day, instead of adding more tasks to it at the end of the day. Multitasking can be great sometimes. But multitasking can't always be proactive. If you're a proactive multitasker, then you're a great person!

Being in a meeting and answering emails is not proactive. Be open to asking for help and support. Go up your chain of command. They can offer you solutions right away, like adding an assistant or assigning your tasks to another person. If not, they can ask for confidential surveys from other leaders to compare and see if there's a bigger issue; it's not just you.

So, ask yourself regularly: did I make any progress today?

Another issue that affects nurse leaders is the lack of training. Training in progressive leadership in nursing, to be more specific. You got here by being a charge nurse, then a nurse manager, and then getting promoted to assistant nurse manager, or Director. But most never received formal training on how to navigate the healthcare system or how to manage finances, productivity, time management, or even Microsoft Excel to make spreadsheets. What they learned about all of this was empirical or they took courses on their own.

Nowadays, that is changing, and some people still mention it in their CVs when applying for jobs. A good example is when asked to share a progress report. Some people spend 30 minutes to create an email with slides, while others spend hours or an entire day to do it. Some days you don't know how to do something or get things, and that is an actual issue for nurse leaders.

A solution would be to have a nurse residency training program, but for leaders. Training before they hit the actual unit. Two to three weeks of training before assuming their roles and increasing their productivity.

Q: What do you think are the major stressors and burnout reasons for leaders?

Mike: Nurses have educational and compliance training responsibilities that can't be done during their shifts or out of their regular schedule because they have childcare issues or a second job. I usually have 100 to 200 employees who report to me. Once, I had 240 employees who reported to me, directly and indirectly. So, to have them all compliance-trained was a real challenge. Chasing people is stressful for leaders. Especially regarding Joint Commission or annual evaluation surveys. Because the compliance guidelines are not being met. It's easy to say, "She's always been non-compliant," or "She doesn't know how to do it." But are we giving that nurse the time to do it?

Some healthcare systems give them 4-6 hours to complete it. However, some of them want them to do the surveys or educational training during their work time. So, if the nurse must go home late or get there early, there will be another big issue around this. So, if you want your workforce to be better, you need to invest in them. Because they can't manage 100 things at the same time. They will be frustrated and burnt out. They can't focus on the one thing you hired them for, which is to take care of patients.

The same goes for charge nurses and nurse managers. They want to make rounds in their units. They want to round patients and have meaningful conversations with the patients and their family members to see how they're doing, but 1,000 phone calls come in, and if there's something they can take care of for that patient, it doesn't happen. That gives me stress as a leader because I know that they don't have enough time to do this or things directly related to their role. It's like when you're a parent. If my kids aren't behaving, I feel bad. If they do well, I do well, and I am happy. If they don't, then I need to look into why. This used to give me panic attacks. So assigning time for those things helps them and our units. Everybody wins. Meeting nurse compliance regulations is important and beneficial to everyone.

Worry, guilt, and a sense of responsibility as a leader is a big deal. You feel like you want to do it for them, but you can't. Your attitude and outlook decide your day, your patient's day, and your unit's day, despite what's going on. It doesn't matter how things are going. A groggy nurse affects my mood, too. Compassion fatigue or secondary stress syndrome is like secondary smoking. It's not me, but I'm still affected and stressed by it. It's a real thing. For example, I am an organized person. When I go and ask someone how they're doing and they respond rudely, I feel bad and stay worried the rest of the day. This happens to everyone at any level. So, the outlook is important. So, you need to learn how to compartmentalize what is personal and what is work-related. You're here for 12 hours; you can't be anywhere else. If you can't separate them, then make a quick phone call, go to the break room, and let what's troubling you go. But don't carry that negativity for your 12 hours.

Outlook and positivity are important because it helps you and everyone around you. The same goes for negativity; it attracts more negativity.

Q: What's the best advice or takeaway you want to give to your colleagues?

Mike: When you're driving to work, what are your thoughts and mood? Is it, "I'm gonna have a good day" or "Man, I don't wanna go there, I hate my job." If this happens, then you're not doing the right job. Maybe there's something wrong with you as a person. Or there's something wrong with the job. The way that you're doing it or the support you're getting.

Look into those three categories.

1. If it's something about you, then yes, go see a counselor or a doctor and get your hormones checked. Or ask your family or friends if they've noticed anything different or strange about you.
2. Job: get a work buddy, talk to your superiors, or find a mentor down the road. Everyone should have one! They can help you manage this in the right way. Just tell them, "I can't do it because it seems like I don't have the joy about my job anymore."
3. Find another job that gives you happiness. Nowadays, we have mental health counselors in almost every healthcare organization. There's also the Employee Absence Program (EAP), which 90% of employees rarely use. It's there for a reason, OSHA enforces it for a reason. There are free counseling and free psychiatric consultations available. Not because you're a psychiatric person but because you need someone to talk to. Someone who can identify your issues and guide you to the steps you can take to find that joy again. If nothing is working for you after trying this, then yes, it's time to find a new job. Don't just quiet quit. It's a new phenomenon. Don't just take time and wait it out. That psychological stress happening in your mind can affect you with a stroke, a heart attack, or many things eventually. Not today, but it will happen to you. So, might as well be happy now, less stressed. Find a job that works well for your mind.

Q: What comes to mind when you hear someone say, "I'm just one person; I can't truly make a change"?

You plant the seeds with your actions. And it's your choice to follow your manager's or leader's steps. Or at least help them reflect on these approaches. I always tell my onboarding managers they have the power in their hands now. You have the power to change at least one person's life.

For example, when someone requests a day off or wants to get approved for an educational course or anything related to management, say yes. There are different things you can do for a person that will make a difference in their life. You might not see it or know it directly. Not everyone has that kind of position, so if you have 100 people under you, you are getting that many chances to change lives, and they can change the lives of the patients they are taking care of. So use that power in a good way. Support and bring up more new leaders. Coach, mentor, and support them.

COMMENT: if you know where to look, there's always an opportunity.

Q: What are you most excited about? What are you looking forward to?

Mike: I am happy about the new structure of the health system. I know that nurse leaders are even happier. The pandemic put nurses in the spotlight, and many understood how valuable and important they are and the struggles they experience. The last time this happened was during the HIV/AIDS outbreak from 1993 to 1995. People were quitting their jobs, and there was instability. It took 30 to 40 years for the healthcare system and the general public to understand what it takes to be a nurse. Because of this, every healthcare system, big or small, has invested, directly or indirectly, in providing more balance to the nurses. And creating more educational programs and mentorships for nurses. So 10 years from now, nursing will be a different profession.

Where people will probably want to work in nursing again. It's slowly happening now. A 30-minute lunch break is not enough now. More rest periods with a massage, aromatherapy, or watching TV after five to six hours and coming back slowly to work. There would be less burnout with more support and resources. So yes, lots of good things are coming to support the nurses' workflow.

[end of interview]

Liz and Mike's insights clarify one thing: we all want to create a culture of care that thrives. This means putting patients first and addressing their full range of needs, from urgent to preventive. We need corporations and top managers to support us. It's possible to deliver high-quality care while keeping healthcare profitable.

They highlight the significant challenges that healthcare leaders face. Handling burnout, keeping up team spirits, and managing the demands of the healthcare system is a lot. Their experiences provide important advice about the tough parts of being a leader. Their stories show why we need to make big changes, give more help, and be kinder in how we run healthcare places. There's a human being in that chair—a person who often receives more complaints than proactive support. Through their experiences, we can better understand the strength, hard work, and dedication needed to lead in this tough field. Their stories show us that, even though the path is hard, leadership has a big impact. It affects patient care and the happiness of healthcare workers. They play an important role in the system.

Next time you find yourself frustrated with your upline, pause, take a deep breath, and get curious. Put yourself in their shoes and identify the challenges they're facing. Then, work together to overcome those challenges and achieve a mutual goal. As someone who has been a leader on several occasions, I know that it is a lonely role. Leaders often face reactive blame and harsh comments from team members who feel their needs aren't being met. While this might be true for some leaders in certain situations, it's not the rule of thumb. Empathy, compassion, and patience can go a long way.

Liz and Mike's stories paint a vivid picture of the challenges and rewards of healthcare leadership. Resilience, empathy, and continuous improvement are key. Their experiences showcase this. These qualities are important for overcoming the field's challenges. Leaders must do more than just manage tasks. They must create an environment where everyone feels supported and valued, themselves included. Letting all workers reach their full potential if they so desire.

Pause and Reflect: Based on the experiences and insights shared by Liz and Mike. How might you approach your interactions with healthcare leaders from now on?

05 Getting started: A glimpse into your journey

All right, this is it! It's time to spill the beans about the evidence-based solutions you can apply daily to be at ease, recharge your energy, and recover properly while at work and during spare time.

When a gymnast is trying to push, fly, and land a technique, they know that improving their stability and having a stronger foundation is key. So learning, repeating, and rehearsing specific movements will fortify the muscles needed for that technique.

Rushing and trying to skip steps won't get her anywhere.

The same principle applies to life. I had to learn to bear the scarcity. To stay stuck in that sticky situation, to become aware of what was actually keeping me there, and to build a strong foundation of wisdom, character, and resilience.

After years of trying hard, analyzing, and working my ass off and nothing fricking changed or improved permanently, no matter what I tried to do, I had no choice but to go within.

When I allowed myself to feel the pain, the struggle, sit with the frustration, the impatience, and the anger, that's when my life consistently took a turn for the better. It wasn't sparks of hope and motivation here and there. I'm talking about life-changing experiences with my health, finances, and relationships.

Day by day, I just sat with my stickiness, so I could learn to be more patient and more tolerant and convince myself that my old ways of approaching and doing were actually what was keeping me tied down more than I thought.

It made me see more clearly that the thoughts, beliefs, and habits were keeping me there in that sticky and uncomfortable situation and accept that it was always about me vs. my beliefs. Not karma, luck, or the universe.

Balance is your new compass

Swimming with the tide is easier and more fun than swimming against the current. The same goes for when your work aligns with your core values. This alignment is especially important in combating burnout. When the demands of the job threaten to overwhelm you, core values can provide clarity and motivation, reminding you why you chose this path. Making it easier to navigate stressful situations without losing sight of your passion and commitment.

Identifying these values starts with introspection—reflecting on what matters to you both personally and professionally. For some, this may be compassion, integrity, and/or advocating for those who can't by themselves. Once identified, these values become a source of strength and direction, your new compass. Helping you stay grounded and focused even in the most trying times. Remaining true to your principles will always nourish you and help you replenish your energy no matter the circumstances.

Navigating Acceptance and Change in Nursing

It's important that as you learn to apply these proven strategies in your life, to be kind, patient, and flexible with yourself. This is not a race to see who reaches full-on Zen mode. It's a new lifestyle where you will incorporate different habits, beliefs, and approaches. There will be days where everything will flow smoothly, others where you will question your sanity and a few more where you simply forget to use these tools, and that is okay!

The difference this time around is that stress won't affect you as much as it has before thus it will be easier for you to prevent or overcome burnout. The best part is that some strategies you will learn in this chapter can be applied anywhere, anytime, even while you are at work. Imagine having a shield that protects you from all the things that trigger you, deplete your energy, or take away your sleep like a thief in the night. So if things are tough and unfair right now in the healthcare field, don't you agree that it's best to have an extra layer of protection until things improve?

Balancing acceptance and change is a delicate dance for nurses on the path to personal growth and burnout recovery. Acceptance involves recognizing and embracing current realities—understanding that some aspects of the job are inherently stressful. This acknowledgment can be freeing, as it removes the burden of fighting against what is. However, true growth comes from identifying areas where change is possible and necessary. This might mean setting stronger boundaries, finding new ways to manage stress or different ways to do your job. The tricky part lies in discerning what to accept and what to change. Too much acceptance can lead to complacency and compassion fatigue, while too much focus on change can lead to frustration. Striking the right balance is key to sustainable growth and recovery.

Recognizing your power and accepting that it's all up to you will take a huge weight off your shoulders because it means you don't have to wait on anyone or anything to improve your life. You have all that you need and always have a choice. I'll say it again, you are prone to make mistakes like us all, so when you set the bar low on your expectations, the journey is more enjoyable. Taking responsibility for your actions without shame or blame is so liberating and opens the doors to exciting new ways of experiencing life. Even if you make a mistake or think that you have failed. I was always looking at what I missed or didn't do right instead of recognizing my accomplishments or all the positive things I had going on for me. If I did, they were short-sighted. Somedays, everything was going well, but a comment someone made about me would throw me off, and I would end up overthinking and feeling awful afterward. But now that I can cultivate patience and curiosity, and I am okay with being vulnerable, things always turn out well. My health and joy are at their best while also being successful financially while doing what I love. I finally accepted that life is meant to be fun!

On that note, let's start with something that we can all relate to. There's a saying that if you do what you love, you'll never work a day in your life. So, if we are so passionate about it, we should do more of it, and everything will simply flow smoothly. If that were true, then why are so many nurses dealing with burnout? Where's the mismatch?

Even if you get to do what you love 100 % of the time, which is rare, even for the most successful people in the world. Most of us get to work on what we are passionate about 80% of the time. The remaining 20% you are doing tasks that are neutral or that you don't enjoy. This means you still need time to rest, recover, and deal with responsibilities. Feeling motivated, creative, and excited are great to experience and fulfilling but sometimes we might not know when to stop. If you don't set healthy boundaries for yourself, you might start feeling pressured, frustrated, or even confused as to why everything is not as easy as you thought it would be. When in reality all you need is a break. This applies to all individuals, but since nursing can be emotionally challenging for many reasons and on so many levels, successful nurses have developed emotional regulation skills, and don't hesitate to seek support when needed. They focus on their mental health, ensuring they have strategies in place to manage stress and prevent emotional exhaustion. This empowers them to navigate the demands of the profession while maintaining their well-being.

The role of our emotions

Our emotions are a life force, influencing our physiology, chemistry, and hormones. They are central to the experience of stress, with cortisol—the stress hormone—being the most affected by our emotions. Emotions propel us to pursue what we want to do by fueling the belief and determination needed to make our dreams happen, even when others say it's impossible.

What we consider positive emotions like happiness, joy, gratitude, care, and compassion are renewing emotions. They replenish our energy levels. And what society considers negative emotions like anger, fear, and frustration are depleting emotions.[33]

Emotions are neither positive nor negative; they're all essential to our humanity. Embracing all emotions is key to healing and avoiding burnout. Thus, we must regulate our emotions. Our mind, like our body, needs regular upkeep. It needs nutrition, sleep, exercise, relaxation, and pleasure. Healthy emotional management can accomplish this.

The most successful people in high-pressure professions keep a steady pace and sustain their success over time because they intentionally make space to tend to their minds and train themselves to be more observant of their thoughts and underlying emotions. It's not because they are always in a good mood or only feel renewing emotions. They are comfortable experiencing both types, sometimes at once, and simply deciding which emotion they want to feel longer and act on. There's a scientific explanation for this.

The brain functions as a pattern identification and matching system.[34] Any input to the brain from your outer and inner environment contributes to the maintenance of these patterns. These continuous inputs eventually become familiar to the brain like our digestive, respiratory, and hormonal rhythms. These familiar patterns help the brain organize perceptions, feelings, and behaviors. So from this baseline, any new experience is compared to what the brain has in its system.

Many of these inputs come from the heart. With every beat, it transmits complex patterns of neurological, hormonal, pressure, and electromagnetic information to the brain and throughout the body. The heart is not simply a pump, it has the most developed communication system to the brain than any other major organ in our body. According to Pribram's theory of emotion, when an input is noticeably different than your baseline, it generates feelings or emotions.

Why is this important?

Because it proves that you can change your baseline. You can train your brain to create new familiar patterns from the new inputs you are consciously providing it with. Eventually, your mind and body will learn to respond differently to stress and not generate depleting emotions.[35] And that's exactly what I'm showing you how to do in this chapter.

The brain automatically strives to maintain a match between familiar mental, emotional, and physical processes and the current state, whether or not it negatively affects your health, well-being, or behavior. The brain doesn't judge; it simply identifies patterns and matches them to its baseline. Your first baseline was created when you were born and during your childhood, depending on the experiences you had growing up and how you learned to respond to challenging or scary situations. Based on this reference, our body activates the stress response and responds to it in the way we have trained it to. So even though we can't eliminate the stress response per se, we can change how our body responds to it by changing our neurological patterns, and hence physically changing our brains. This is called neuroplasticity and there have been many research studies about it.[36]

That's why anxiety, depression, and other symptomatic behaviors, thoughts, or emotions can become the familiar baseline, the reference pattern for many years, or an individual's entire life. The person doesn't feel happy or well. It becomes part of his identity, forever self-perpetuating and self-reinforcing even if he doesn't want to be this way. For some, these are the folks that we see have challenging lifestyles but do nothing about it, even if they don't like living this way. But when the person becomes aware of this and creates a conscious change in his patterns, things will take a 180-degree turn for the better. Now, as an adult, you can re-write your story, generate a new baseline, and create a life aligned with who you truly are and how you wish to live it. Isn't that exciting and amazing?

Through emotional refocusing and restructuring, instead of having a big release of adrenaline along with emotions like fear, anger, revenge, or getting defensive. We can respond to stress with increased alertness and more thoughts around it to predict and analyze what is happening around us coherently.

Learning to establish and sustain new patterns requires practice, consistency, and patience while your brain restructures this process. Eventually, maladaptive patterns related to stress are replaced by healthier physiological, emotional, cognitive, and behavioral patterns and they become the new familiar way of being, and you will think, behave, and feel like it by default.

A few years ago, I was at my son's baseball game when I suddenly heard someone scream, "Help! Is there a nurse or doctor around?" I jumped up from my bench and ran to find a man on the ground with a dislocated knee. After I stabilized him, called 911, and made sure he was safely transported, I went back to watch my son's game. Within minutes, I started shaking all over and felt nauseated. It was the adrenaline release! Since leaving the bedside, it was the first time in five years I had to attend to someone in need in a public place. I took deep, slow breaths and told myself everything was all right. The person would be okay, and so would I. It's shocking to realize how numb we become while working in a hospital. In over 25 years as a nurse, I had experienced nothing similar because my body was in survival mode 95% of the time. That adrenaline rush was part of my bread and butter.

Installing your new software

Remember, we are all born with the hardware: our brain and our neural connections. We covered this in Chapter One. Yet, some mental states, like our beliefs and perspectives, can make it challenging. Our mindset is our software. There is no problem with the hardware; we can change our ways anytime, but there are many problems with the software. Perception can greatly affect our experience of stress.

To install new mental habits, we need to establish a new baseline that the brain recognizes as familiar. This requires retraining our bodies through a multifaceted approach. These efforts focus on helping you identify patterns in your behavior and emotional responses, which is a key step in developing emotional regulation skills. This process also lays the groundwork for exploring coping strategies and creating action plans to manage those reactions more effectively.

That night, after the baseball game, I had another A-Ha moment. In my 30s, I had difficulty feeling emotions like happiness, joy, and euphoria. Even when receiving the best news or having life-changing experiences like getting married, I felt happy but not ecstatic. I wondered if something was wrong with me or if I was being ungrateful. It seemed like a big deal, yet my reaction was just, "Yeah, alright, thank you." That night, I saw the connection. I had trained myself to numb my emotions so well, especially as a nurse working in Intensive Care, that my body was still programmed to respond this way. Since then, whenever I'm doing a task, I take a deep breath and set the intention: "I choose to feel happy at this moment as I'm working on this document" or "Giovanna, you did so good today, and tomorrow will be even better!." When I'm moody or frustrated, I do something similar: I pause, take three deep breaths, and talk to myself, "I know I'm cranky because I'm tired. When I take a short break and grab a healthy snack, I know I'll feel better. So, for now, I acknowledge you, frustration, but you're just an emotion. You are not who I am. So I will continue to feel you, and at the same time, I choose to be patient with myself."

This process helps me immensely. Instead of venting or taking out my frustration on my husband or kids, I can manage my stress effectively. It's a win-win: my health stays intact, and no one must deal with me when I'm having a bad day.

Resisting change

Most of us are familiar with the mental and logical approaches to solving our problems. But I'm certain that you have experienced more than once, like myself, that sometimes you will want something different even if you don't exactly know what that is. You just intuitively know that you're missing something.

Change is part of life, it's inevitable, but the process can be comfortable or rough. When you integrate more parts of your true self in this process, the faster and more easily it will happen. That's why I use a holistic approach, accessing the wisdom of my body, mind, and spirit. This approach, combined with the standard mental approach, is effective as it helps us look at patterns in our behaviors and how to plan. More energy flows when different parts of yourself are aligned, making it easier to achieve what you subconsciously believe.

Think of yourself as a river. When all the tributaries—the different parts of your life and self—flow in the same direction, the river becomes stronger. Similarly, when all aspects of your identity and values are aligned, your energy and focus are amplified, letting you navigate life's challenges with greater ease and confidence.

To access your body, you can go for a walk outdoors or even around your house while checking in with the sensations in your body. Most pain and medical conditions have an emotional root. For example, shoulder pain can be related to our ability to carry out experiences in life joyously, stomach issues might stem from dread or fear of the new, and jaw pain can signify resentment or anger. By doing this, you are engaging in two processes instead of thinking about it.[37]

To access your spirit, take a couple of deep breaths (direct connection with the autonomic processes) and find a comfortable position. Then ask yourself:

- What brings me great joy?
- When do I feel most alive?
- What helps me be more patient and compassionate?
- What are my greatest accomplishments in life so far?
- What makes my career meaningful?
- Who do I admire? What is that person's life purpose?
- Which leaders inspire me?
- How can I be more like them?
- Who or what makes me feel appreciated and needed? Who seeks my services while compensating me fairly?
- How can I create more experiences like that?

- What would I stand for if I knew no one would judge me and I couldn't fail?
- Could this be a right career, wrong job type of situation?
- What would my ideal job and lifestyle look like?
- If my life had no limits and I could have it all and do whatever I wanted, what would I have and do? How would my life change?

According to Gallup, only 20% of the world's population is passionate about what they do.[38] It's time to make the shift. It all starts with looking for deeper significance in everyday experiences, even at work. It's about finding lessons, insights, or personal growth opportunities in each situation, no matter how routine or challenging. This approach helps you stay engaged and motivated by seeing the value in everything you do.

Meanwhile, if the job doesn't fit, the short-term solution is to keep your eyes on the prize. Decide to create your vision and an informed action plan.

When your inner and outer worlds are in sync, everything clicks into place. It cuts down on false starts because you're more in tune with what's true for you. The decisions you make and the actions you take lead to lasting change.

The change process is different for everyone, and it's definitely not linear. It's more like a roller coaster. You enter the theme park (contemplation), you decide to go for it (decision), and while in line, you feel excited and nervous, questioning your choice (preparation). So many what ifs. Once you're on the ride (action), you know there's no going back, so you simply enjoy it, even if you scream the whole way (maintenance). You took a chance, even though you weren't 100% sure, and it turned out to be fun.

The same applies to this journey of recovering from burnout and making changes. It's important for you to acknowledge which stage of change you are in and do things related to that stage. Some people want to jump from the start line to the finish line without preparing ahead of time or contemplating all that needs to happen so they can get to the finish line. That's when doubt, frustration, disbelief, and hopelessness can take over.

It's normal if one part of us wants to change while another doesn't. The resistance to change might be due to being busy and not wanting to add more things to your list. We usually focus on our responsibilities, and not on investing more time in research, contemplating, or planning because we believe that we are too busy or too tired to do it. We might even fantasize about a spontaneous change out of the blue! This usually happens when we don't get enough rest or appreciation from others for our efforts. We are so busy taking care of others that there's no energy or time left for you. I've seen this show up as an obstacle in my client's change process 90% of the time.

So, if this is you, and you don't want to spend time planning, ask yourself what needs to happen so time for you is part of your weekly activities. A suggestion might be to simply pick one to four hours in the week for you. Don't do anything for your loved ones or your family, it's all about you. You don't need to plan anything for those hours either unless you want to. Do what you feel like during those hours that is healthy and nourishing. Then and only then you can do something for others during the rest of that day you are off. Once your loved ones see the benefits of this change they will encourage you to keep doing it. Some might not support your decisions and that's when you will know who you should spend more time with.

The resistance could also be due to fear. This often happens when we start making changes and overpromising. Because changes that can't be sustained lead to another false start.

Choosing small steps or easy/fun strategies will help you feel accomplished and see fear as an ally. Fear turns into excitement because you realize that fear is actually helping you move slowly but effectively toward your goal. You're doing something new that is taking you out of your comfort zone.

- *I don't have an issue. It would be easy if I had all the time and money in the world, but my responsibilities and work are always getting in the way.*
- *Maybe it is an issue, but not a big one. So, if I go for a massage or a vacation, everything will be better when I get back. If that doesn't work, I'll get a new job.*
- *I have an issue, but I can't make any progress due to our healthcare system anyway. So why bother? I just don't have the willpower. When I tried before, it didn't work, so why would I think I could do it now?*

If these thoughts keep coming up when you wish things were different, then it's time to raise your consciousness. By identifying the dominant thoughts and the emotions tied to them, you can get to the root cause of why you don't believe that change is an option right now. Holistic coaching sessions are wonderful when you find yourself in similar situations, but for now, you can start by asking yourself:

- What is the one thing I need most right now?
- What is my worst fear about it? What's the worst thing that could happen?
- Is this fear true or an old assumption? Did I hear it from my parents or teachers?
- Is it true for me now?
- Would I be better off if I dropped that belief?

These questions will help you reset parts of your software if you integrate them with the strategies outlined below. Remember, no one thinks in your mind but you.

Emotional Regulation

I used to hate crying when I was younger. It made me feel weak and embarrassed. Whenever I felt afraid or angry, I thought I was not a good girl or that something was wrong with me and that I should behave differently. In the Western world, we often accept renewing emotions but don't fully express them, while we usually reject depleting emotions. Admitting that we're not okay can be challenging for many.

I learned the hard way that suppressing our emotions can lead to more significant issues eventually. It's a silent type of stress that can cause numbness and anger and eventually lead to an outburst. On the flip side, recognizing depleting emotions makes it easier to understand their sources. By addressing these emotions constructively rather than letting them fester, they can be transformed into opportunities for growth and self-improvement.

Embracing and expressing all emotions is important for emotional stability and well-being. Both renewing and depleting emotions are necessary, and achieving a balance between them is essential. As my favorite mentor says, positive emotions generate positive energy that can enhance one's life, while negative emotions, if not managed well, can drain energy and hinder personal growth. By becoming aware of the emotions experienced, one gains better control over life. Taking responsibility for and expressing emotions allows for more authenticity, and people will love you more for that.[39]

Start by becoming aware of your emotions. This means recognizing what you're feeling and understanding the triggers behind those feelings.

1. What situations, people, or events usually trigger strong emotions?
2. What emotions do you find most challenging to manage, and why?
3. When experiencing a strong emotion, what physical sensations or thoughts go along with it?
4. When you can better identify those depleting emotions and attitudes commonly called stress, it will be easier to replace them with the ones that facilitate renewal. How can you anticipate and prepare for these triggers?
5. Can you recall a recent situation where you felt overwhelmed but you managed it well? What happened, and how did you respond?
6. How can you apply those strategies to the current situation that triggers you?
7. What positive coping mechanisms would you like to try or develop further?
8. How do you typically express your emotions, and how does this impact your relationships?
9. How does your emotional state affect your decision-making and interactions with others?
10. What support systems or resources can you access to help with emotional regulation?
11. What small, realistic goals can you set to improve your emotional regulation?

Reflect on these questions regularly to increase self-awareness, identify emotional patterns, and develop practical strategies for managing emotions more effectively. Keep these questions handy throughout your journey.

On those days when something is eating you up, and there will be a few of those in this journey, look at it from a distance as if it were happening to someone else. This perspective can help give the inner critic a new role without silencing it. Acknowledge what is being experienced, name the emotions without feeling embarrassed or guilty, and decide which direction you want to go:

- Do you want to ignore why you feel this way and let yourself get swept up by your emotions?
- Or do you want to verify if what you are feeling is true or something that you believe you should feel based on experiences? Take responsibility without shame or blame. Remind yourself that you are human, experiencing a human moment and that you always get to choose how to respond to it.

Develop Coping Strategies

Learn and practice techniques to manage your emotions and regulate your nervous system. They will help you give your body a taste of what feeling safe, relaxed, and at ease feels like as you do them. So the more you do them with intention, the easier it will be for your brain to create a new baseline with new patterns on how to respond to stressful circumstances with a newly regulated nervous system.

Starting with just five minutes a day, using any of these tools can lift your spirits and clarify how to handle emotional challenges.

Remember, taking small, actionable steps with low expectations makes the process more enjoyable and sustainable.

a) Deep breathing exercises are one of my favorites because it's one of the most effective ways to reduce stress by activating the body's relaxation response. It helps you slow down and stop the automatic responses and any impulsive actions you might take. It is free, quick, and powerful and you can do it anytime. Some techniques can be done even as you're talking to someone and they will never know. Making it a convenient tool for managing stress and promoting overall well-being in the heat of the moment by telling your body to use more of your parasympathetic responses instead of the usual sympathetic response of flight or fight.

The simple act of changing your breathing pattern to make it slower and deeper can help shift energy. Deep breathing and closed-eye visualization – techniques that mindfulness meditation usually employs – also boost alpha brain waves. It can help you release tension, think of a new option, not react impulsively, sleep better, or integrate information differently.

Here are some of the most effective techniques:

Box Breathing Also known as square breathing, this technique involves inhaling for 4 seconds, holding the breath for 4 seconds, exhaling for 4 seconds, and holding the breath again for 4 seconds. Think of it like the four corners of a square, with each phase of the breath representing one corner. This cycle can be repeated multiple times and helps to calm the nervous system.

4-7-8 Breathing Developed by Dr. Andrew Weil, this exercise involves inhaling for a count of 4, holding the breath for a count of 7, and exhaling for a count of 8. This method is said to help reduce anxiety and promote better sleep.

Visualization Breathing Combine deep breathing with visualization by imagining a peaceful scene or a soothing color filling your body as you inhale, and stress or tension leaving your body as you exhale. This can enhance the calming effects of deep breathing. Each color has a special meaning and powerful effect on people. With my intuitive coaching clients, I tell them which color to focus on based on what they are going through at that moment and they find it very beneficial.

I saved the best for last, **the Quick Coherence technique from HeartMath Institute.** It is a simple yet powerful method designed to help you quickly shift into a state of balance and harmony, reducing stress and promoting overall well-being. It can be used to calm reactive emotions, reduce feelings of worry and fear, reduce feelings of overwhelm and stress, and quiet an overactive mind. It involves two main steps: Heart-Focused Breathing and activating a positive feeling.

Step 1: Heart-Focused Breathing

1. **Focus Your Attention on Your Heart:** Sit comfortably and gently place your attention on the area around your heart. Imagine your breath is flowing in and out of your heart or chest area.
2. **Breathe Slowly and Deeply**: Inhale slowly and deeply through your nose to a count of five, and then exhale slowly and deeply through your mouth to a count of five. Maintain a steady, smooth rhythm. Continue this for a few breaths.

Step 2: Activate a Positive Feeling

1. **Recall a Positive Experience:** While continuing to breathe deeply, recall a time when you felt good inside. This could be a feeling of appreciation, care, or love for someone or

something in your life, such as a loved one, a pet, a special place, or an enjoyable activity.

2. **Feel the Positive Emotion**: Try to re-experience that positive feeling. Focus on it and let it fill your heart and mind. This helps to amplify the effects of Heart-Focused Breathing and shifts your emotional state to one that is more coherent and balanced.

If you enjoyed this technique, HeartMath has many more free resources online.

b) Meditation can seem mysterious, woo-woo, or even contradictory to some religions, but its benefits are well-documented and accessible to anyone. As with any meditation practice, the purpose isn't just to spend time disconnected from your problems, your past or future, only to open your eyes and go back to your reality, your habits, your not-so-healthy coping mechanisms, and reacting the same way to stress. It's essentially a way to train your mind, similar to how physical exercise trains your body.

Regular meditation can reduce stress, improve focus, and promote emotional health. Since it increases alpha waves, your relaxation brain waves, and reduces beta waves, the brain waves of active thought and learning. Studies show it can lower blood pressure, enhance sleep quality, and boost your immune system. It's like giving your mind a reset button so you understand yourself better and be able to move through the world in a way that serves you better. Helping you to feel more balanced and present in everyday life even if nothing outside you has changed. Letting you pause, take a nice deep breath, and respond in a coherent way rather than react in the same old way. It can also help you experience different states of consciousness, build more character, coming from wisdom or compassion, and uncover a sense of origin, and reconnect with a deeper sense of life and spirituality, which is the goal of most religions and traditions.[40] Prayer and contemplation can also help you.

If you are new to meditation, think you can't do it, or tried it but didn't get it, I invite you to explore it with these tips.

1. **Be Gentle with Yourself:** It's normal for your mind to wander. When it does, gently bring your focus back to your breath or your chosen point of concentration without judgment. The goal is not to quiet the mind completely but to become aware of your thoughts and your body's responses as if you were an observer. Be at peace with whatever arises. The harder you try to quiet your mind, the harder it will be to reach deeper and more beneficial levels of consciousness. The more you allow whatever thoughts, emotions, or sensations to arise during your practice without reacting to it, the more interesting, fun, and beneficial your meditation will be.
2. **Create a Comfortable Space:** Find a quiet and comfortable place where you won't be disturbed. It doesn't have to be elaborate, just a spot where you feel at ease.
3. **Focus on Your Breath:** Use your breath as an anchor. Pay attention to the sensation of breathing in and out. This helps to keep you grounded and present.
4. **Try Different Techniques:** there are various meditation practices like sitting down, lying down, walking, or with movement like Tai Chi. There are also different styles, such as silent meditation, guided meditation, mindfulness, loving-kindness, or body scan. Ask yourself, what kind of focus helps you relax, find peace, or discover answers to your questions?

   If you know which ones keep doing them consistently. If you don't, try a few different ones and see which one resonates the most with you.

5. **Use several resources:** Especially initially, guided meditations can provide structure and help you stay on track. You can also go to in-person classes, workshops, retreats, or even online programs. I learned to meditate using Dr. Joe Dispenza's teachings. I liked his ways because he explained it from a scientific and medical perspective so it resonated with my medical background.
6. **Be Consistent:** Regular practice is more beneficial than occasional long sessions. Try to meditate at the same time each day to build a habit. Once you have made it part of your daily self-care activities you can alternate which times of the day you do it.
7. **Set an Intention:** Before you start, set a clear intention for your practice. It could be to relax, to become more aware of your thoughts, to connect with your true self, to feel more love or simply to enjoy some quiet time.
8. **Notice Your Body:** Pay attention to how your body feels. You can do a quick body scan, noticing any areas of tension and letting them relax. You can even talk to the body part that is tense or uncomfortable and lovingly tell it that all is well and that it's okay to relax.
9. **Use Technology Wisely:** There are many apps and online resources that offer guided meditations, timers, and tips for beginners. These can be helpful tools. Some biofeedback equipment can help you understand how you shift your state of mind depending on what you are thinking. You can get out of a calm state and have a stressful response by having negative thoughts. The same goes for positive thoughts. The choice is always yours.
10. **Journal Your Experience:** Before and after meditating, take a few minutes to write down your experiences and any insights. For example, what you are thinking, and how you are feeling physically and emotionally before you meditate

and afterward. This can help you track your progress and reflect on your journey.

Remember, meditation is a personal practice, and there is no one-size-fits-all approach. Find what works best for you, and be patient with yourself as you develop your practice. I used to experience so much anxiety and high levels of stress it took me 3 years to go deeper within while I meditated. My tendency to control, over-analyze, and predict the outcome didn't help much either. But once I did, it changed my life in so many aspects. Some people can achieve this with just one meditation or in a short period. The difference lies in how open you are to stepping out of your comfort zone with curiosity and excitement.

c) Progressive muscle relaxation (PMR) is a technique used to reduce stress and promote relaxation by systematically tensing and then relaxing different muscle groups in the body. The idea is to increase awareness of physical tension and teach the body how to release it. PMR can be effective for reducing stress, improving sleep, and enhancing overall relaxation.

1. Choose a comfortable, quiet place where you won't be disturbed. You can sit or lie down. Make sure your body is supported, in a relaxed position, and that you are comfortable.
2. Take a few deep breaths to calm yourself and bring your attention to your body.
3. Start with One Muscle Group, like your feet or hands. Tense the muscles in that area as tightly as you can (without straining) for about 5-10 seconds.
4. Release and Relax: Slowly release the tension and let the muscles relax completely. Focus on the sensation of relaxation and the difference between tension and relaxation.

5. Move to the Next Muscle Group: Progressively work your way up through different muscle groups (calves, thighs, abdomen, chest, arms, shoulders, neck, and face), following the same process of tensing and relaxing. If you find any specific areas where you feel tension or have difficulty, you can spend extra time on those areas.

   Regular practice helps in becoming more attuned to your body's tension and relaxation responses. Aim to practice PMR daily or as needed for stress relief.

d) Grounding exercises are a technique for you to firmly anchor yourself in the present moment by reorienting you to the here and now and to reality. Grounding exercises are helpful when having a bad day or dealing with a lot of stress, overwhelming feelings, stuck on a strong emotion, and/or intense anxiety. It's a self-soothing skill that you can also use when you want to concentrate better on a specific task and not be distracted by distressing memories, thoughts, or feelings.

Steps:

1. Stand up, ideally over grass and barefoot, but it's not mandatory.
2. Take some deep breaths, and spend a few breaths imagining that your feet are like the roots of a tree. Feel connected to the ground, even if you are inside a building.
3. Visualize the energy of anger, fear, or frustration gently leaving your body, from your head down to your feet, and returning it to Earth. Let it go with gratitude and ease as you exhale.
4. When you inhale, imagine renewing, fresh energy coming up from your feet, to your heart, then to your head, and up to the skies.
5. Keep repeating for as long as you like.

6. If a specific feeling arises during this grounding exercise, you can sit with it for as long as you like to see what else comes up, or you can choose to shift that feeling right away. Ask yourself, 'What is the thought behind this emotion? How can I change that thought or feeling right now?' Trust whatever your intuition suggests in that moment. The more in touch you are with your emotions and the present moment, the easier it will be to listen to your intuition and act on it without hesitation.
7. You can use this technique while at work, even if you are sitting down in a meeting, before starting your shift, or when your coworkers are speaking negatively about something. You can even say in your mind, "This is not who I am, this is not my story, I'm not speaking defeat," so I'm lovingly releasing this back to Earth or whatever mantra or affirmation resonates the most with you.
8. Another activity you can try when you are calm so it is easier to ground yourself next time you are stressed is to breathe slower and deeper than usual, then use your five senses (sight, sound, smell, taste, and touch) and notice something with each of them. This simple yet powerful action of becoming aware with one sense at a time is beneficial.

e) Engaging in hobbies and activities you enjoy

- Spend time outdoors, at least 5 minutes each day. Soaking up some sun, feeling the breeze, and being surrounded by nature always provides a calming and replenishing effect on us. It's part of our DNA to be outdoors.
- Journaling or having an honest conversation with yourself and expressing what your heart wants at that moment.

- Daily gratitude practice: give thanks when you wake up before getting out of bed for all the things you are grateful for. Your pillow and a good night's sleep count!
- Listening to your favorite uplifting music while cleaning, driving, or cooking.

f) Choose your food wisely Your mood is influenced by the food you eat. There's a strong gut-brain connection. Food is a gift from nature and a special one because it's the only materialized source of energy we can directly receive. Think about it: most food is solid, liquid, or something in between, and when we digest it, we break it down into essential nutrients and energy that fuel our bodies and support our well-being. Your brain is made of billions of molecules, most of which come from what you eat. This means you can improve the components in your brain by making healthier food choices and taking the proper supplements for your needs.[41]

People's issues around food and eating are often the expression of a larger need for nourishment. Whether it's physical, emotional, mental or spiritual nourishment. It can also be related to the Giving and Receiving cycle that I explained in earlier chapters, there could be an issue with resting, receiving, or elimination and releasing.[42]

I'm not a nutritionist, so I don't provide dietary recommendations, but want to share you can start by noticing how you feel before and after you eat a meal. Keep track of which food energized you and kept you full and which ones only made you more hungry and crave more things and if any of them changed your mood. By tracking, you will intuitively know what's best for your body.[43]

If you want to go deeper into your nourishment issues or how you eat, you can start by asking yourself:

- How would you describe your intake of all kinds of things in relation to your letting go of all things? Are they equal? Do you take more in than let go or vice versa?
- How is your activity and rest balance? Is one more common than the other?
- Classify your food as nourishing or non-nourishing—there's no such thing as bad food.

g) Exercising for stress relief when fatigued or burnt out. Exercise can be a powerful tool for stress relief. It might seem counterintuitive to work out when you're exhausted, but even gentle movement can boost your energy levels and improve your mood.

- **Walking:** A brisk walk outdoors can clear your mind and provide a change of scenery.
- **Yoga:** Gentle yoga stretches can help release tension and calm your mind. You can even add some fascia and lymphatic draining moves into it.
- **Stretching:** Simple stretching exercises can alleviate physical stress and refresh your body.
- **Tai Chi:** This slow, flowing martial art promotes relaxation and mental focus.
- **Swimming:** Light swimming or floating in water can be soothing and rejuvenating.

These activities don't require intense effort but can significantly help reduce stress, recharge energy levels, and rejuvenate the spirit. Intense exercises like running, especially during high-stress levels or burnout, might not be advisable. Although running is considered eustress and can aid in improvement, during burnout, it might lead some individuals to push their bodies and minds too hard. When you're burnt out, you don't need any additional pressure. The focus should be on resetting, relaxing, and recharging. Gentler forms of exercise might be more beneficial in such cases.

There is nothing magical about breaking paradigms and overcoming past situations that no longer serve you; it requires hard work and consistency. Tolerance and respect are essential for everyone, including your own body. Pay attention to its feedback, how do you feel after eating, exercising, and sleeping? It may take time to feel rested and relaxed, but improvements should be noticeable, such as:

- feeling less anxious
- having fewer worrisome thoughts
- being in a better mood more often
- showing more tolerance towards others
- being motivated to continue improving
- feeling optimistic about the future
- experiencing less drain from issues at work

These subtle but significant signs indicate progress toward recovery from the physical, mental, and emotional exhaustion endured.

For extra reassurance and because many of us are fascinated by science, let's dive into how brainwaves impact our mood and mental state, helping us either relax or boost our energy. By gently guiding these brainwaves, we can steer ourselves toward the mental state we desire. It's like having a remote control for your mental well-being.

For example, focused attention is linked to increased beta waves, associated with alertness, the use of our senses, and concentrated mental states. This can sometimes lead to overanalyzing and racing thoughts. By focusing on the present moment, cultivating greater awareness of sensations, and paying attention to your breath, you can enhance brain activity related to attention while also benefiting from alpha waves, which promote relaxation and creativity.

Beta waves act like your brain's cheerleaders, keeping you sharp and on point, essential for tasks requiring concentration and problem-solving.[44] Alpha waves help you relax, spark creativity, and boost mood by increasing serotonin. Plus, high-intensity workouts can boost alpha waves, giving you a post-exercise glow and mental uplift.[45]

If you want to get even more science-y, studies have found an increase in gray matter volume (GMV) and gray matter density (GMD) in various brain regions of individuals who practice Mindfulness-Based Stress Reduction strategies. Humans need gray matter to learn and remember, make decisions, and regulate emotions.[46] Mindfulness isn't just about chilling out: it's about changing your brain and even your IQ! For deeper states of focus and meditation, theta waves become prominent, reflecting the profound impact mindfulness can have on brain activity.

Wearables and neurofeedback devices can help train brainwaves, or you can use brainwave entrainment techniques like binaural beats[47] to sync brainwaves with external stimuli. If beats aren't your thing, there are music services designed to enhance specific brainwaves.

Incorporating these strategies can actively guide brainwaves to achieve the mental state you want, improving overall well-being and cognitive functions. So, explore the strategies previously mentioned. Your brain will thank you, and you'll feel amazing!

Remember, setting healthy boundaries is not selfish; it's selfless. It helps you be more effective and better able to support others. Sometimes, boundaries are necessary to counteract the stubborn drive that pushes you to keep going, neglecting the need to pause and take care of yourself. Resting doesn't just mean taking a physical break; it can also include practices like deep breathing exercises on the go, solitude, or listening to your favorite tunes.

As you finish this chapter, reflect on your journey. What strategies have resonated with you? How can these insights enhance your work and personal life? Jot down thoughts or plan to try one new approach this week. Remember, it's the small, consistent steps that lead to meaningful change. Keep a journal to track your progress and revisit these strategies as needed.

Curious about living a healed life? Let's turn the page to the last chapter.

06 What does a healed life look like?

A healed life doesn't guarantee that everything will always unfold exactly as you wish, but it means you can navigate whatever comes your way with inner calm and strength. It's about embracing a state where the mind can breathe and the heart can rest, free from the pull of extremes. Imagine floating effortlessly on calm waters, anchored in peace and stability, with no waves to disrupt your serenity. In this space, you're simply present, finding clarity in the quiet flow of your inner balance. Trusting in divine timing allows you to embrace each moment with a balanced heart and mind. Whether things unfold differently or take longer than expected, you remain anchored in the belief that everything is happening for your highest good. When you embrace this, intellectual fear will no longer stop you from pursuing what burns in your heart.

As a nurse, this balance allows you to care for others while safeguarding your well-being. A healed life means supporting others without sacrificing your health. Even on the toughest days, you can maintain fulfillment and joy in your work by setting healthy boundaries and prioritizing self-care. You can face the emotional and physical demands of the job with strength, knowing how to recharge your energy. Some days, it will be easier to let go of triggers; on others, it might be more challenging. Yet, you remain optimistic, trusting that everything is part of a phase in your life, unfolding for a reason—even if it's hard to understand or painful now.

Your Life Purpose

Accomplishing a fulfilling life is easier when you understand and stay focused on your life purpose. Keeping your eyes on the prize makes sure every decision and action aligns with your goals, helps you overcome obstacles, including those uncomfortable responsibilities or insecurities. It's common to lose sight of your goals amidst daily challenges, but regularly reminding yourself of what you want in life and focusing on it can help keep you on track. Everything else is secondary.

Meaningful work is important for a fulfilling life. Recent research shows that how people perceive their workload affects burnout more than the number of hours worked.

Working to improve yourself, your career, and your relationships begins with envisioning what you want most. Consider these questions:

- If you could choose any future, what would it be?
- What would you do if you believed you could achieve anything?
- What would a passionate and fulfilling career look like?
- What makes you feel you're not (fill in the blank) _____ enough to pursue it? Where did this belief originate?

How can you start?

Think about small changes you can make this week to get you to do what you love, even without immediate financial rewards. Start part-time, preparing for a full-time pursuit.

You don't need to dedicate all your time and energy right away, but remember your goals and take small, consistent steps toward them. Use your natural interests, talents, and personality to bring joy and uplift others.

Focus on smaller victories that will slowly lead you to your ultimate goal. Tackling small tasks is less daunting than facing a large goal without a plan. Push your boundaries by doing something that scares you each day. If you keep doing more of the same, you will continue to get the same result. Like when you were learning to drive, start with small steps, and work up to conquering bigger fears. This process will help you grow stronger and more fearless.

If you're struggling with ideas, take a break to rest and recharge. When you're calm, you're more likely to listen with your heart and let ideas flow effortlessly.

Embracing Mistakes and Turning Them into Success

Mistakes are a part of life, especially in high-pressure jobs like nursing. I've made my share of mistakes in both nursing and life. These mistakes can evoke feelings of guilt and shame that linger for years.

Replaying the same thoughts and feelings drains our energy. It shifts our perspective and shapes our behavior, often without us realizing it. Over time, this becomes part of our identity.

As a neuroscience research nurse, I've seen this pattern in thousands of people. But here's the truth: mistakes aren't the enemy – they're teachers.

Here are three powerful mindset shifts to turn setbacks into growth opportunities:

1. **The Brain Learns From Mistakes—Challenges Help Us Grow:** View mistakes as chances to learn. They reveal your strengths and areas for improvement.
2. **Separate Your Self-Worth from Outcomes:** You're more than a single success or failure.
3. **Embrace Curiosity:** Instead of fearing the unknown, ask yourself, "What can this teach me?"

Embracing mistakes makes you stronger and more adaptable. It boosts your confidence in your decisions and in taking action.

When you make a mistake, ask yourself:

- What circumstances led to the mistake? Common causes include rushing, fatigue, multitasking, and stress. Also, a lack of preparation, pressure to please, or acting out of routine can cause it.
- Did fatigue, stress, or overconfidence contribute?
- Did a lack of planning or communication cause it?
- How did you feel at the time of the mistake?
- What did you learn from the experience?
- What strengths have you shown in the past that can help you overcome this challenge?

You've likely noticed that, after a few days, sometimes the situation wasn't as bad as it first seemed. Or that the outcome led to something positive in an unforeseen way.

Your commitment to growth and doing better each day defines your excellence as a nurse, not perfection.

When self-doubt creeps in, focus on your abilities rather than your perceived shortcomings. Don't fear failure – it's a life lesson. You'll never know your full potential if you don't push yourself to grow.

Challenge your limiting beliefs. Imagine yourself being joyful and aligned with your purpose. Stay focused on what truly matters—it all begins with a single thought!

When anxiety keeps showing up

Picture this: you've had a good month overall. But then, without warning, you wake up in the middle of the night. As you try to drift back to sleep, your mind starts replaying everything you did—or didn't do—over the past month. Before you know it, you're caught in a full-blown 2 a.m. panic.

Sound familiar?

Difficulty sleeping and late-night worrying are all too common for healthcare workers. It's something most of us experience at some point. Anxiety shows up uninvited, and guilt often tags along for the ride. But here's the truth: lying awake and stressing over what's done—or left undone—won't fix the situation or help you get the rest you need.

When you have a healed life, you can quickly turn this around. You understand that you always have the power to put yourself in control of your thoughts and actions. By stepping back from your worst fears and making sure you control your emotional response — and not the other way around — it's possible to dismiss those negative thoughts and actually get some sleep at night.

This is why learning to release anxiety is so important for us nurses. We are so focused on the anxiety and frustration we fail to recognize the silver linings, even when they are right in front of us. Learning how to calm your fears and feel confident about your choices is a matter of education, action, and respect.

So next time anxiety shows up, acknowledge it and give thanks to your body because it's asking you to pay attention to something. Then, reflect on the feeling. Is it real? What are the sponsoring thoughts behind it? If you are in bed, tell yourself that now is the time to rest and that you will think about this tomorrow. Take a few deep breaths and focus on how good that feels instead of forcing yourself to go back to sleep.

Here are additional steps you can take to regain control and stop anxious thought patterns as you are creating new habits and a better lifestyle:

1. **Focus on the positive:** recognizing and appreciating your strengths and current positive relationships with others. Remembering a time when you overcame a challenge and felt accomplished and proud.
2. **Self-checkups:** Asking yourself if what you are thinking is true or an assumption helps you identify problem areas and calm your fears. You might be picturing a worst-case scenario to something that might never happen because you are comparing this situation to a past experience, where the circumstances and people involved were different. This means that the outcome could also be different if you're open to it.

3. **Banish shame or guilt:** remember that as nurses, we have a lot of responsibilities and unrealistic expectations imposed on us. So, even if you didn't get everything done when you wanted, you still did a lot for your patients, co-workers, and yourself. You did the best you could with the resources you had at that moment.
4. **Stop comparing yourself:** everyone else is dealing with their issues, even if it seems like they have it all figured out or life is easier for them. Trying to measure up often makes you feel like you aren't where you should be and adds to your overall stress level and anxiety based on mere assumptions.
5. **We usually fear what we don't understand.** If fear of the unknown causes you to stress, turn those unknowns into knowns. You can do this by emotionally regulating and practicing how to change your thought patterns and your nervous system response on demand with the strategies I shared with you in the previous chapter.
6. **Express your feelings healthily daily, don't bottle them up.** Acknowledging your feelings without judgment can help reduce their intensity.

Feeling more anxious when changing an old behavior

Has this ever happened to you? You start a new eating plan and exercise routine, and things are going well—you're seeing results and feeling good about your progress. Yet, some days, you feel a strong urge to slip back into old habits. Or maybe you notice a surge of anxiety but can't quite pinpoint the reason why.

Changing an old behavior can often be a daunting task. It's common to feel a surge of anxiety when attempting to break away from familiar routines. This anxiety may stem from uncertainty, fear of the unknown, or the comfort that old habits provide. For many, there's also a strong pull to revert to previous behaviors, especially when under stress or faced with challenges. This can make the process of change feel overwhelming and discouraging.

Here are tips on how to resist the pull of old habits

1. **Acknowledge Your Feelings:** It's important to recognize that feeling anxious or tempted to return to old habits is normal.
2. **Set Clear, Achievable Goals:** Start with small, specific changes rather than attempting a complete overhaul all at once. This makes the process more manageable and less intimidating.
3. **Develop a Plan for Challenges:** Identify potential triggers or situations that may tempt you to revert to old habits. Develop strategies in advance to handle these moments, such as deep breathing exercises, mindfulness techniques, or seeking support from your network.
4. **Create a Support System:** Surround yourself with supportive friends or family for accountability or encouragement. If you feel alone or different because no one around you is applying this type of learning or aren't taking proactive action to improve their health and life, see it as an opportunity to lead by example. They will soon start noticing that you aren't speaking or behaving like you used to and they will get curious. If they are good friends they will support you and might even join you in creating a new lifestyle that works for them and not to please other's expectations.
5. **Celebrate Small Wins:** Recognize and celebrate each small step you take towards change to boost your confidence and motivation.

6. **Practice Self-Compassion:** Be kind to yourself during this process. Change is difficult, and setbacks are a natural part of the journey. Instead of being critical, use setbacks as learning opportunities.

As you find proactive ways to stay on top of your responsibilities, to-do list, and emotional responses you may find that the anxious feeling that comes when you go to bed dissipates in favor of control and confidence.

If the anxiety or pull towards old habits is overwhelming, consider seeking help from a therapist or counselor. They can provide tools and strategies to navigate these challenges effectively.

Feeling stuck due to others

When everybody else is feeling stressed and anxious, that's the time for you to show courage. Start telling the truth, and be authentic.

It's natural to feel stuck or hurt when others don't get you or support your dreams. If they let you down or betray your trust, it can be even more challenging, but there are steps you can take to move forward. Start by acknowledging your feelings and giving yourself permission to grieve the loss or betrayal. It's essential to set boundaries to protect your well-being and focus on self-care. Lastly, focus on what you can control—your actions and responses—and remember that healing takes time.

You can easily say, "I'm feeling angry, what that person did really hurt me. It might take me some time to flush this pain out of my system, but I choose to see this as a lesson to be learned or a moment of growth for me. Since it's a temporary thing, I prefer to focus on doing things that nourish me and not spend any more time or energy on that situation." Even if you have to catch yourself 10-20 times a day to emotionally regulate and do some of your favorite coping techniques.

Say this: "This is my anger, frustration, and pain, and I am releasing it calmly." Practice helps you feel more emotionally organized every time a challenge arises.

You will want to take action, set healthy boundaries, and do what is necessary to address how that person hurt you. But focus on processing that painful situation clearly and thoughtfully, as it will help you become stronger and wiser.

Catching yourself

You might catch yourself when something is stopping you, like if someone offers you a great opportunity, but you are hesitant. You feel bad without even trying it. So ask yourself: why do I feel this way? Where does this come from? Trace it back to your childhood and see when you believed that you weren't worthy of receiving.

Accept that what you inherited isn't your fault or your parent's fault. They were only doing their best with what they had at that moment. It's no one's fault. It needed the happen even if you never get to understand why.

If something keeps showing up in your life and is stressing you out, then it's time to look at it from a distance, as if you were a third person watching yourself. Stress highlights where life problems are hiding.

Healing comes from understanding. Even if you can't heal all your hurts at once, after healing things, you feel more courageous and ready to take more risks. Be it starting a new business, finding a partner, or going on a trip. You will feel more energized and more hopeful for your future. What is waiting for you?

If you don't take the risk you might never find out.

For a long time, the thought of the future filled me with fear. This fear kept me stuck, unable to pursue my aspirations. While fear offered a sense of security, I now realize it was actually limiting me. I needed to trust that life was guiding me and be open to releasing the old stories I held onto. I had to have faith that better things were waiting for me. Once I embraced this trust, the uncertainty cleared away. Suddenly, I learned of the countless opportunities surrounding me. Adopting this new perspective let me explore all the incredible possibilities life had in store. None of these dreams would have come to fruition had I remained fearful and small. Now, it's your turn to do the same—release the fear, trust in the journey, and watch as your life transforms.

What's next?

Life is an ever-evolving journey, and change is a constant companion. Embrace the power of reflection and intuition, and regularly evaluate how your strategies are guiding you. Become more self-aware by exploring aspects of yourself with curiosity rather than judgement. This way, you can ensure they align with your life purpose and growth efforts.

Be open to adjusting your approach as you learn more about what helps you manage your emotions effectively.

Create your own opportunities to grow. Always keep learning and reinventing yourself in a fun way: work on skills like empathy, self-regulation, and effective communication. This can involve reading books, attending workshops, finding a mentor/coach, or even seeking feedback from others about how you handle emotions.

You could sabotage these exciting and potentially life-changing opportunities that will start showing up for you if you aren't mentally prepared for change, which is why you need to be open and willing for any experience that comes your way.

You've already done the hard work; now it's time for you to receive. You are worthy!

Tap into your genuine passions, skills, and intuition. By doing so, you'll not only find happiness but also inspire those around you. Now is the time to embrace your uniqueness, speak your truth, and live with intention. Burn bright from within, not out, and let your inner light guide you toward a truly fulfilled life.

Book references and links

1 HeartMath Institute. (n.d.). HeartMath Interventions Online Certification Program for Health Professionals. Retrieved August 4, 2024, from https://store.heartmath.com/heartmath-interventions-certification-program-for-health-professionals/

2 https://www.drlarosa.com/blog/burnout

3 Alonso Puig, M. (2024). *Resetea Tu Mente: Descubre de Lo Que Eres Capaz / Reset Your Mind: Discover What You're Capable of.* Planeta Publishing Corporation.

4 Alonso Puig, M. (2024). *Resetea Tu Mente: Descubre de Lo Que Eres Capaz / Reset Your Mind: Discover What You're Capable of.* Planeta Publishing Corporation.

5 https://www.drlarosa.com/blog/burnout

6 Fenmi, L., Ph.D., & Robbins, J. (2007). *The Open Focus Brain: Harnessing the power of attention to heal mind and body.* Trumpeter Books.

7 https://www.drlarosa.com/blog/burnout

8 Cannon, W. B. (1932). The wisdom of the body. New York: Norton.

9 https://www.health.harvard.edu/staying-healthy/understanding-the-stress-response

10 Alonso Puig, M. (2024). *Resetea Tu Mente: Descubre de Lo Que Eres Capaz / Reset Your Mind: Discover What You're Capable of.* Planeta Publishing Corporation.

11 Kleijweg, Jeroen & Verbraak, Marc & Van Dijk, Maarten. (2013). The Clinical Utility of the Maslach Burnout Inventory in a Clinical Population. Psychological assessment. 25. 10.1037/a0031334.

12 Anna Sjörs Dahlman, Ingibjörg H. Jonsdottir, Caroline Hansson, Chapter 6 - The hypothalamus–pituitary–adrenal axis and the autonomic nervous system in burnout, Editor(s): Dick F. Swaab, Ruud M. Buijs, Felix Kreier, Paul J. Lucassen, Ahmad Salehi, Handbook of Clinical Neurology, Elsevier, Volume 182, 2021, Pages 83-94, ISSN 0072-9752. (Bianchi et al., 2015). (https://www.sciencedirect.com/handbook/handbook-of-clinical-neurology) https://s100.copyright.com/AppDispatchServlet#formTop

13 https://www.providencetreatment.com/addiction-blog/the-12-stages-of-burnout-identification-prevention-treatment/

14 https://www.drlarosa.com/blog/burnout

15 Amilhon, B., Ducharme, G., Jackson, J., Goutagny, R., Williams, S. (2020). Theta Rhythm in Hippocampus and Cognition. In: Dang-Vu, T., Courtemanche, R. (eds) Neuronal Oscillations of Wakefulness and Sleep. Springer, New York, NY. https://doi.org/10.1007/978-1-0716-0653-7_2

16 Nuñez, A., & Buño, W. (2021). The Theta Rhythm of the Hippocampus: From Neuronal and Circuit Mechanisms to Behavior. *Frontiers in Cellular Neuroscience*, *15*, 649262. https://doi.org/10.3389/fncel.2021.649262

17 Nuñez, A., & Buño, W. (2021). The Theta Rhythm of the Hippocampus: From Neuronal and Circuit Mechanisms to Behavior. *Frontiers in Cellular Neuroscience*, *15*, 649262. https://doi.org/10.3389/fncel.2021.649262

18 Alonso Puig, M. (2024). *Resetea Tu Mente: Descubre de Lo Que Eres Capaz / Reset Your Mind: Discover What You're Capable of.* Planeta Publishing Corporation.

19 https://www.chiefhealthcareexecutive.com/view/reducing-burnout-in-doctors-focus-on-fixing-the-workplace-not-the-worker

20 https://www.who.int/news/item/28-05-2019-burn-out-an-occupational-phenomenon-international-classification-of-diseases

21 Cannon, W. B. (1932). The wisdom of the body. New York: Norton.

22 Cannon, W. B. (1932). The wisdom of the body. New York: Norton.

23 HeartMath Institute. (n.d.). HeartMath Interventions Online Certification Program for Health Professionals. Retrieved August 4, 2024, from https://store.heartmath.com/heartmath-interventions-certification-program-for-health-professionals/

24 HeartMath Institute. (n.d.). HeartMath Interventions Online Certification Program for Health Professionals. Retrieved August 4, 2024, from https://store.heartmath.com/heartmath-interventions-certification-program-for-health-professionals/

25 LeDoux, J., The Emotional Brain: The Mysterious Underpinnings of Emotional Life. 1996, New York: Simon and Schuster.

26 https://vcahospitals.com/know-your-pet/signs-your-dog-is-stressed-and-how-to-relieve-it

27 Pichère, P., & Cadiat, A.-C. (2015). Maslow's hierarchy of needs. Lemaitre.

28 McCraty, R., Heart-brain neurodynamics. The making of emotions. 2003, Boulder Creek, CA: HeartMath Research Center, Institute of HeartMath, Publication No. 03-015

29 McCraty, R., Heart-brain neurodynamics. The making of emotions. 2003, Boulder Creek, CA: HeartMath Research Center, Institute of HeartMath, Publication No. 03-015

30 Golmaryami, F.N., Frick, P.J., Hemphill, S.A. et al. The Social, Behavioral, and Emotional Correlates of Bullying and Victimization in a School-Based Sample. J Abnorm Child Psychol 44, 381–391 (2016). https://doi.org/10.1007/s10802-015-9994-x

31 https://link.springer.com/article/10.1007/s10802-015-9994-x

32 https://www.psychologytoday.com/us/basics/imposter-syndrome#:~:text=People%20who%20struggle%20with%20imposter,discover%20the%20truth%20about%20them

33 McCraty, R. and D. Childre, The appreciative heart: The psychophysiology of positive emotions and optimal functioning. Boulder Creek, CA: HeartMath Research Center, Institute of HeartMath, Publication No. 02-026, 2002.

34 Pribram, K.H., Emotions: A neurobehavioral analysis, in Approaches to Emotion, K.R. Scherer and P. Ekman, Editors. 1984. Erlbaum: Hillsdale, NJ.

35 McCraty, R., and D. Tomasino, The coherent heart: Heart-brain interactions, psychophysiological coherence, and the emergence of system-wide order. 2006, Boulder Creek, CA: HeartMath Research Center, Institute of HeartMath, Publication No. 06-022

36 https://www.health.harvard.edu/blog/brain-plasticity-in-drug-addiction-burden-and-benefit-2020062620479#:~:text=Neuroplasticity%20refers%20to%20our%20brain's,levels%20in%20response%20to%20experience.

37 Hay, L. (1988). *Heal Your Body: The Mental Causes for Physical Illness and the Metaphysical Way to Overcome Them*. Hay House. (Hay, 1988, #)

38 https://www.gallup.com/workplace/394871/employee-wellbeing-starts-work.aspx

39 Honda, K. (2019). *Happy money: The Japanese art of making peace with your money*. Penguin Life.

40 Bark, L., & Bark Phd, L. (2011). *The Wisdom of the Whole: Coaching for Joy, Health, and Success*. CreateSpace Independent Publishing Platform. P285

41 Hanson, R., & Mendius, R. (2009). *Buddha's Brain: The Practical Neuroscience of Happiness, Love & Wisdom*. New Harbinger Publications.

42 Bark, L., & Bark Phd, L. (2011). *The Wisdom of the Whole: Coaching for Joy, Health, and Success*. CreateSpace Independent Publishing Platform. P 263

43 Harvard Health Publishing. "Can Mindfulness Change Your Brain?" *Harvard Health Blog*, 13 May 2021, www.health.harvard.edu/blog/can-mindfulness-change-your-brain-202105132455. Accessed 3 August 2024.

44 Lustenberger, C., Boyle, M. R., Foulser, A. A., Mellin, J. M., & Fröhlich, F. (2015). Functional role of frontal alpha oscillations in creativity. *Cortex, 67*, 74-82. https://doi.org/10.1016/j.cortex.2015.03.012

45 Hölzel, B. K., Carmody, J., Vangel, M., Congleton, C., Yerramsetti, S. M., Gard, T., & Lazar, S. W. (2011). Mindfulness practice leads to increases in regional brain gray matter density. *Psychiatry Research*, *191*(1), 36. https://doi.org/10.1016/j.pscychresns.2010.08.006

46 Jefferson Health. "How to Manipulate Brain Waves for a Better Mental State." *Nexus*, 10 March 2022, nexus.jefferson.edu/science-and-technology/how-to-manipulate-brain-waves-for-a-better-mental-state/. Accessed 3 August 2024.

47 Gallup. (2022). *Employee wellbeing starts at work*. Gallup. https://www.gallup.com/workplace/394871/employee-wellbeing-starts-work.aspx

Made in the USA
Columbia, SC
02 May 2025